D0877674

Maternal-Neonatal Nursing

Third Edition

Lynne Hutnik Conrad, RN,C, MSN

Nursing Program Director
Maternal-Child Health
Allegheny University Hospitals
Elkins Park, Pennsylvania

Springhouse Corporation
Springhouse, Pennsylvania

Staff

Executive Director
Matthew Cahill

Editorial Director
June Norris

Art Director
John Hubbard

Managing Editor
David Moreau

Acquisitions Editors
Patricia Kardish Fischer, RN, BSN;
Louise Quinn

Clinical Consultant
Maryann Foley, RN, BSN

Editor
Ellen Newman

Copy Editors
Cynthia Breuninger (manager),
Christine Cunniffe, Brenna Mayer,
Pamela Wingrod

Designers
Arlene Putterman (associate art director), Lesley Weissman-Cook (book designer), Diane Armento-Feliz, Joseph J. Clark, Jacalyn Facciolo, Linda Franklin, Donald G. Knauss, Kaaren Mitchel, Matie Patterson, Mary Stangl

Typographers
Diane Paluba (manager), Joyce Rossi Biletz, Phyllis Marron, Valerie Rosenberger

Production Coordinator
Margaret Rastiello

Administrative Assistants
Beverly Lane, Mary Madden, Jeanne Napier

Manufacturing
Debbie Meiris (director), Pat Dorshaw (manager), Anna Brindisi, T.A. Landis

For those organizations that have been granted a license by CCC, a separate system of payment has been arranged. The fee code for users of the Transactional Reporting Service is: 0874348609/96 $00.00 + $.75.

Printed in the United States of America.

SNMN3-020298

℞ A member of the Reed Elsevier plc group

Library of Congress Cataloging-in-Publication Data
Conrad, Lynne Hutnik.
   Maternal-neonatal nursing / Lynne Hutnik Conrad. —
3rd ed.
     p. cm. — (Springhouse Notes)
   Includes bibliographical references and index.
   1. Maternity nursing. 2. Infants (Newborn) —
Diseases — Nursing.
   I. Title. II. Series.
   [DNLM: 1. Maternal-Child Nursing — outlines.
   2. Neonatology — nurses' instruction. 3. Neonatology —
outlines. WY 18.2 C754m 1997]
RG951.C668 1997
610.73'678—dc20
DNLM/DLC for Library of Congress   96-29145
ISBN 0-87434-860-9 (alk. paper)   CIP

Contents

Advisory Board and Reviewers

How to Use
Springhouse Notes

Springhouse Notes is a multi-volume study guide series developed especially for nursing students. Each volume provides essential course material in an outline format, enabling the student to review information efficiently.

Special features appear in every chapter to make information accessible and easy to remember. **Learning objectives** encourage the student to evaluate knowledge before and after study. **Chapter overview** highlights the chapter's major concepts. Within the outlined text, key points are highlighted in shaded blocks to facilitate a quick review of critical information. Key points may include cardinal signs and symptoms, current theories, important steps in a nursing procedure, critical assessment findings, crucial nursing interventions, or successful therapies and treatments. **Points to remember** summarize each chapter's major themes. **Study questions** then offer another opportunity to review material and assess knowledge gained before moving on to new information. **Critical thinking and application exercises** conclude each chapter, challenging students to expand on knowledge gained.

Other features appear throughout the book to facilitate learning: **Teaching tips** highlight key areas to address with patient teaching. **Clinical alerts** point out essential information on how to provide safe, effective care. **Decision trees** promote critical thinking. Difficult, frequently used, or sometimes misunderstood terms are indicated by SMALL CAPITAL LETTERS in the outline and defined in the glossary, Appendix A; answers to the study questions appear in Appendix B. Finally, a brand-new Windows-based software program (see diskette on inside back cover) poses 100 multiple-choice questions in random or sequential order to assess your knowledge.

The Springhouse Notes volumes are designed as learning tools, not as primary information sources. When read conscientiously as a supplement to class attendance and textbook reading, Springhouse Notes can enhance understanding and help improve test scores and final grades.

CHAPTER

Overview of Maternal-Neonatal Nursing

LEARNING OBJECTIVES

After studying this chapter, you should be able to:

♦ Discuss current legal and ethical issues in maternal-neonatal nursing.

♦ Describe the structure and function of families in present-day society.

♦ Describe various roles for maternal-neonatal nurses.

♦ Define the goals of maternal-neonatal nursing.

CHAPTER OVERVIEW

Maternity-neonatal nurses assume a variety of roles and functions in caring for the patient and her family. In certain instances, the functions performed are dependent on the nurse's level of education. An understanding of the make-up and functioning of the family plays a vital role in helping the nurse deliver family-centered care. Even though the structure of the family has changed and technological advances have affected this area over the years, nurses working in this field are responsible for providing comprehensive, ethical, and legal care to the pregnant mother, her fetus, and family.

◆ I. Maternal-neonatal nursing

A. General information

1. The goal of maternal-neonatal nursing is to provide comprehensive, family-centered care to the pregnant patient and her fetus or neonate during the antepartum, intrapartum, and postpartum periods

2. Maternal-neonatal nurses practice in a variety of settings. These may include:
   a. Community-based health centers
   b. Private doctor offices
   c. Hospital clinics
   d. Acute-care hospitals
   e. Maternity hospitals
   f. Birthing centers
   g. The home

B. Nursing roles and functions

1. Nurses involved in maternal-neonatal nursing assume a variety of roles. These may include:
   a. Care provider
   b. Educator
   c. Advocate
   d. Counselor

2. The functions involved for each of these roles is dependent on the nurse's level of education

3. Registered Nurse (RN) is a graduate of an accredited nursing program who
   a. Has passed the NCLEX-RN examination
   b. Is licensed by the state
   c. Plays a vital role in providing direct patient care, meeting the educational needs of the patient and her family, and functioning as an advocate and counselor

4. Certified Nurse Midwife is an RN who has received advanced education at the Masters level or by certification
   a. Independently cares for the low-risk obstetrical patient throughout her pregnancy
   b. Is licensed to deliver the infant

5. Nurse Practitioner is an RN who has received advanced education at the Masters level or through certification
   a. Performs in an expanded, advanced practice role
   b. Obtains histories, performs physicals, and manages care throughout pregnancy in consultation with the doctor

6. Clinical Nurse Specialist is an RN who has received education at the Master's level
   a. Focuses on health promotion, parent teaching, direct nursing care, and research activities
   b. May serve as a consultant to RNs working in the maternal-neonatal field

♦ II. Family-centered care

A. General information
   1. Definition of family
      a. Group of two or more persons related by blood, marriage, or adoption residing together (U.S. Bureau of Census)
      b. Group of persons united by blood, marriage, or adoption who have a common residence for some part of their lives
   2. Family structure
      a. Evolved over the years from the traditional nuclear family
      b. Other family structures include: single-parent, step-parent, blended, cohabitation, communal, and extended
   3. Family functions
      a. No matter the family structure, the primary function of a family is to meet the physical, psychosocial, and educational needs of its members
      b. Physical needs are met through food, shelter, clothing
      c. Psychosocial and educational needs are met as members are instructed in the customs, culture, and religious beliefs and traditions of the family

B. Family influences on pregnancy
   1. Influencing factors
      a. Factors can influence the family's response to the pregnancy
      b. These include:
         (1) Maternal age
         (2) Cultural beliefs and practices related to pregnancy
         (3) Whether pregnancy planned or not
         (4) Family structure and functioning
         (5) Social and economic resources
         (6) Presence, age, and health status of other family members
         (7) Maternal medical and obstetrical history
   2. Implications for nursing
      a. Assessment of each family member's roles and functions
      b. Effect of each member's roles and functions on the other members
      c. Assessment of health beliefs, practices, and resources
      d. Impact of factors on childbearing and family

e. Priority and goal setting to provide individualized care based on the family's needs

◆ III. Ethical and legal issues

A. General information
1. Great technological advances have been made in the areas of reproductive technologies and genetic research
2. This has also created many ethical and legal issues
3. Prenatal testing can provide information regarding gender, congenital abnormalities, and chromosomal defects
4. While this knowledge can help the parents and health care team prepare for the infant, some people fear this knowledge may be used incorrectly. For example,
   a. What if a woman decides to terminate a pregnancy because she is displeased with the fetus' sex?
   b. Will genetic engineering lead to the creation of only "desirable" individuals?
5. The maternal-neonatal nurse must be familiar with these issues and explore her own beliefs in order to present a nonjudgmental attitude.

B. Standards of care
1. Standards of care are guidelines that are based upon scientific principles and provide guidance when providing health care
2. Guidelines upon which these standards of care are developed are set by an accrediting agency (such as the Joint Commission on Accreditation of Healthcare Organizations) and based on the scope of practice as defined by the state's nurse practice act
3. Facilities must meet the agency's minimum standards in order to be accredited
4. Nurses are required to observe at least the minimum standard of care

C. Patient's rights
1. Unless an acute medical emergency prevents the patient from actively participating, the pregnant woman has the right to participate in decisions involving her own health and the health of her fetus
2. In addition to the American Hospital Association's "Patient's Bill of Rights," "The Pregnant Patient's Bill of Rights" explains the specific rights of the pregnant patient

D. Ethical and legal issues
1. INFORMED CONSENT
   a. Prior to treatment, diagnostic procedures, or experimental therapy, the patient must be informed of the reasons for the treatment as well as possible side effects and alternative treatments

b. The doctor must obtain the signed consent

c. The nurse assures it in the patient's chart before the procedure is performed

2. Abortion

   a. Although abortions are constitutionally legal, abortion remains an emotionally charged topic

   b. The obstetrical nurse must examine her personal beliefs and present a nonjudgmental attitude to the patient

3. In vitro fertilization (IVF)

   a. With IVF, the ovum is fertilized outside the body and then reimplanted into the uterus

   b. While this procedure has allowed infertile couples to have a child, there are concerns that it is unnatural and questions regarding the fertilized ova that are not implanted

4. Surrogacy

   a. A surrogate mother carries a fetus for another couple with the expectation the newborn will be adopted by that couple

   b. Questions have evolved over the surrogate mother's legal rights to the infant

5. Fetal tissue research

   a. Fetal tissue has helped in scientific research

   b. There are concerns whether the number of abortions will increase in response to the need for tissue, and whether this is an ethical use of human tissue

6. Eugenics and gene manipulation

   a. Gene therapy can help in the prevention and management of different disorders

   b. Questions arise surrounding the ability to create "desirable" individuals, leading to a "perfect" population

7. High-risk neonate treatment

   a. Medical advances improved survival rates for high-risk neonates

   b. There are concerns regarding the physical, psychosocial, and economic costs

POINTS TO REMEMBER

♦ Nurses working in maternal-neonatal nursing can assume a variety of roles and functions.

♦ The concept of the nuclear family has been replaced with various structures.

♦ Ethical and legal issues have resulted from advances in technology.

♦ Adherence to standards of care and supporting a patient's rights are key to providing ethical and legal maternal-neonatal nursing care. The nurse must present a nonjudgmental attitude when caring for patients.

STUDY QUESTIONS

To evaluate your understanding of this chapter, answer the following questions in the space provided; then compare your responses with the correct answers in Appendix B, page 172.

1. How has the family structure changed within the last 20 years? _____

_____

_____

2. What are three factors that can influence a family's response to pregnancy?

_____

_____

3. What are three practice settings for the maternal-neonatal nurse? _____

_____

_____

4. What is the role of the nurse when dealing with an ethical issue? _____

_____

_____

CRITICAL THINKING AND APPLICATION EXERCISES

1. Follow a Clinical Nurse Specialist for a day. Prepare an oral presentation to your fellow classmates detailing the roles and functions that you observed.

2. Interview a patient and her family. Determine the family structure and the roles and functions of each member.

3. Pick an ethical or legal issue involved in maternal-neonatal nursing. Prepare a debate arguing both sides of the issue.

2

Structure and Function of the Reproductive Organs

CHAPTER OVERVIEW

Knowledge of the structure and function of the male and female reproductive systems is essential for understanding the processes involved with childbearing. Hormones occurring throughout the female reproductive cycle prepare the uterus for pregnancy. Male and female accessory glands also play a key role in this area.

♦ I. Female reproductive system

A. External genitalia
   1. Mons pubis
      a. Provides an adipose cushion over the anterior symphysis pubis
      b. Protects the pelvic bones
      c. Contributes to rounded contour of the female body
   2. Labia majora
      a. Consist of two folds of tissue that converge at the mons pubis and extend down to the posterior commissure
      b. Consist of connective tissue, elastic fibers, veins, and sebaceous glands
      c. Protect the components of the vulval cleft
   3. Labia minora
      a. Located within the labia majora
      b. Consist of connective tissue, sebaceous and sweat glands, nonstriated muscle fibers, nerve endings, and blood vessels
      c. Unite to form the fourchette, the vaginal vestibule
      d. Lubricate the vulva, adding to sexual enjoyment and providing bactericidal protection
   4. Clitoris
      a. Located in the anterior portion of the vulva, just above the urethral opening
      b. Is made up of erectile tissue, nerves, and blood vessels
      c. Consists of the glans, body, and two crura
      d. Homologous to the penis
      e. Provides sexual pleasure
   5. Vaginal vestibule
      a. Is the tissue extending from the clitoris to the posterior fourchette
      b. Consists of the vaginal orifice, the hymen, the fossa navicularis, and Bartholin's glands
         (1) The hymen is a thin, vascularized mucous membrane at the vaginal orifice
         (2) The fossa navicularis is a depressed area between the hymen and fourchette
         (3) Bartholin's glands are two bean-shaped glands on either side of the vagina; they secrete mucus during sexual stimulation
   6. Perineal body—area between the vagina and the anus; the site of episiotomy during childbirth
   7. Urethral meatus—located ⅜″ to 1″ (1 to 2.5 cm) below the clitoris
   8. Paraurethral glands (Skene's glands)
      a. Are located immediately inside the urethral meatus
      b. Produce mucus

Female external genitalia

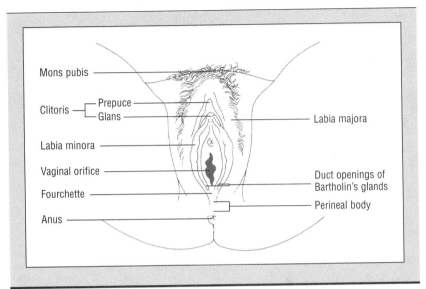

Mons pubis

Clitoris — Prepuce / Glans

Labia minora

Vaginal orifice

Fourchette

Anus

Labia majora

Duct openings of Bartholin's glands

Perineal body

B. Internal genitalia
  1. Vagina
     a. Is the vascularized musculomembranous tube that extends from the external genitals to the uterus
     b. Functions as the copulatory and parturient passage
     c. Acts as excretory duct of uterus for menses and other secretions
  2. Uterus
     a. Is a hollow, pear-shaped muscular organ divided by a slight constriction (isthmus) into an upper portion (body or corpus) and a lower portion (cervix); the body or corpus has three layers
        (1) PERIMETRIUM
        (2) MYOMETRIUM
        (3) ENDOMETRIUM
     b. Provides an environment for fetal growth and development
     c. Receives support from broad, round, uterosacral ligaments
  3. Fallopian tubes
     a. Are about 4¾″ (12 cm) long, consist of four layers (peritoneal, subserous, muscular, and mucous), and are divided into four portions (interstitial, isthmus, ampulla, and fimbria)
     b. Transport ovum from the ovary to the uterus

Female internal genitalia and related structures

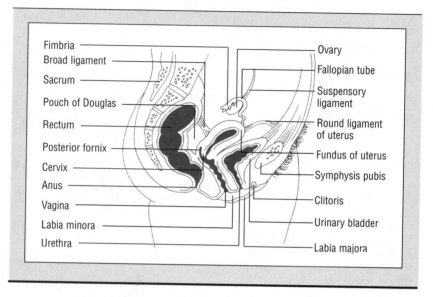

Fimbria
Broad ligament
Sacrum
Pouch of Douglas
Rectum
Posterior fornix
Cervix
Anus
Vagina
Labia minora
Urethra

Ovary
Fallopian tube
Suspensory ligament
Round ligament of uterus
Fundus of uterus
Symphysis pubis
Clitoris
Urinary bladder
Labia majora

    c. Provide a nourishing environment for zygotes

    d. Serve as the site of fertilization

  4. Ovaries

    a. Are two almond-shaped glandular structures on either side of the uterus, below and behind the fallopian tubes

    b. Produce sex hormones (estrogen, progesterone, androgen)

    c. Serve as the site of ovulation

♦ II. Female accessory glands: Breasts

A. Consist of glandular, fibrous, and adipose tissue

B. Grow and develop from stimulation of secretions from the hypothalamus, anterior pituitary, and ovaries

C. Provide nourishment to the infant and transfer maternal antibodies during breast-feeding

D. Enhance sexual pleasure

♦ III. Female reproductive cycle

A. Menstrual phase (days 1 through 5 of the menstrual cycle)

  1. Estrogen and progesterone levels decrease

  2. FOLLICLE-STIMULATING HORMONE (FSH) levels rise, and steady levels of LUTEINIZING HORMONE (LH) initiate estrogen secretion by the ovary

  3. Menstrual flow begins

B. Proliferative (follicular) phase (days 6 through 13)
   1. Estrogen production increases, leading to proliferation of endometrium and myometrium in preparation for possible implantation
   2. Follicle secretes estradiol
   3. FSH stimulates graafian follicle
   4. FSH production decreases before ovulation (approximately day 14)

C. Secretory (luteal) phase (days 14 through 25)
   1. The CORPUS LUTEUM forms under the influence of LH
   2. Estrogen and progesterone production increase
   3. The endometrium is prepared for implantation of fertilized ovum

D. Ischemic phase (days 26 through 28)
   1. The corpus luteum degenerates if conception does not occur
   2. Estrogen and progesterone levels decline if conception does not occur

◆ IV. Male reproductive system

A. External genitalia
   1. Penis
      a. Has three layers of erectile tissue—two corpora cavernosa and one corpus spongiosum
      b. Consists of the body (shaft) and glans
      c. Deposits spermatozoa in the female reproductive tract
      d. Contains sensory nerve endings that provide sexual pleasure
   2. Scrotum
      a. Is a pouch-like structure composed of skin, fascial connective tissue, and smooth muscle fibers
      b. Contains two lateral compartments that house the testes and related structures
      c. Protects the testes and spermatozoa from high body temperature

B. Internal genitalia
   1. Testes
      a. Are two oval-shaped glandular organs inside the scrotum
      b. Produce spermatozoa
      c. Produce testosterone, the primary male sex hormone, and other androgens
   2. Epididymides
      a. Serve as the initial section of the testes' excretory duct system
      b. Store spermatozoa as they mature and become motile
   3. Vas deferens
      a. Connects the epididymal lumen and the prostatic urethra
      b. Serves as a conduit for spermatozoa

Male reproductive system and related structures

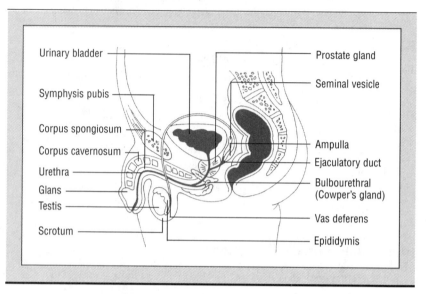

Urinary bladder
Symphysis pubis
Corpus spongiosum
Corpus cavernosum
Urethra
Glans
Testis
Scrotum
Prostate gland
Seminal vesicle
Ampulla
Ejaculatory duct
Bulbourethral (Cowper's gland)
Vas deferens
Epididymis

4. Ejaculatory ducts
    a. Located between the seminal vesicles and the urethra
    b. Serve as passageways for SEMEN and seminal fluid
5. Urethra
    a. Extends from the bladder through the penis to the external urethral opening
    b. Serves as the excretory duct for urine and semen

♦ V. Male accessory glands

A. Seminal vesicles
    1. Are two pouch-like structures between the bladder and the rectum
    2. Secrete a viscous fluid that aids in spermatozoa motility and metabolism
B. Prostate gland
    1. Consists of glandular and muscular tissue
    2. Is located just below the bladder
    3. Is considered homologous to Skene's glands in females
    4. Produces an alkaline fluid that enhances spermatozoa motility and lubricates the urethra during sexual activity (the urethra runs through the center of the prostate)
C. Bulbourethral glands (Cowper's glands)
    1. Are two pea-sized glands opening into posterior portion of urethra
    2. Secrete a thick alkaline fluid that neutralizes acidic secretions in the female reproductive tract, thus prolonging spermatozoa survival

POINTS TO REMEMBER

◆ Fertilization occurs within the fallopian tubes.

◆ The female reproductive cycle is marked by cyclic hormonal changes.

◆ The primary male sex hormone is testosterone.

◆ Spermatozoa survival and motility in the female reproductive tract depend on the alkaline secretions of the male accessory sex glands.

STUDY QUESTIONS

To evaluate your understanding of this chapter, answer the following questions in the space provided; then compare your responses with the correct answers in Appendix B, page 172.

1. Which reproductive structure is formed from the joining of the labia minora?

_____

_____

2. Which three ligaments provide support to the uterus? _____

_____

_____

3. What are the four phases of the female reproductive cycle?_____

_____

_____

CRITICAL THINKING AND APPLICATION EXERCISES

1. Prepare an oral presentation to a group of adolescent girls describing the female reproductive cycle.

2. Diagram the hormonal feedback system involved with the female reproductive system.

3

Fetal Growth and Development

CHAPTER OVERVIEW

Intrauterine development begins with gametogenesis and progresses to the term fetus. Fetal growth and development occur over a period of 40 weeks, with the development of specialized structures and events along the way. Certain structures, including fetal membranes, umbilical cord, placenta, and amniotic fluid are unique to the fetus. Additional specialized structures develop that differentiate fetal circulation from extrauterine circulation.

◆ I. Genetic components

A. General information
   1. Chromosomes are structures within the cell nuclei that contain an individual's genetic make-up
   2. The normal number of chromosomes is 46 — 23 from each parent
   3. Cellular multiplication occurs when the zygote undergoes *mitosis,* dividing into two cells, four cells, and so on
      a. These cells, called *blastomeres,* eventually form the *morula,* a solid ball of cells
      b. After the morula enters the uterus, a cavity forms within the dividing cells, thus changing the morula into a blastocyst

B. Gametogenesis
   1. *Gametogenesis* refers to the production of specialized sex cells, called *gametes*
      a. The male gamete (spermatozoon) is produced in the seminiferous tubules of the testes during spermatogenesis
      b. The female gamete, or OVUM, is produced in the graafian follicle of the ovary during oogenesis
   2. As gametes mature, the number of chromosomes they contain is halved (through meiosis) from 46 to 23

◆ II. Conception

A. General information
   1. Fertilization occurs with the fusion of a spermatozoon and an ovum (oocyte) in the ampulla of the fallopian tube
   2. The fertilized egg is called a *zygote*
   3. The diploid number of chromosomes (44 autosomes and 2 sex chromosomes) is restored when the zygote is formed
      a. A male zygote is formed if the ovum is fertilized by a spermatozoon carrying a Y chromosome
      b. A female zygote is formed if the ovum is fertilized by a spermatozoon carrying an X chromosome

B. Implantation
   1. *Implantation* occurs when the cellular wall of the blastocyst (the trophoblast) implants itself in the endometrium of the anterior or posterior fundal region, about 7 to 9 days after fertilization
   2. Primary villi appear within weeks after implantation
   3. After implantation, the endometrium is called the decidua

C. Placentation
   1. In *placentation,* the chorionic villi invade the decidua
   2. This becomes the fetal portion of the future placenta

♦ **III. Fetal structures and development**
   A. Fetal membranes
      1. The chorion is the fetal membrane closest to the uterine wall; it gives rise to the placenta
      2. The amnion is the thin, but tough, inner fetal membrane that lines the amniotic sac

   B. Embryonic germ layers
      1. *Ectoderm* generates the epidermis, nervous system, pituitary gland, salivary glands, optic lens, lining of the lower portion of the anal canal, hair, and tooth enamel
      2. *Endoderm* generates the epithelial lining of the larynx, trachea, bladder, urethra, prostate gland, auditory canal, liver, pancreas, and alimentary canal
      3. *Mesoderm* generates the connective and sclerous tissues; blood and the vascular system; musculature; teeth (except enamel); mesothelial lining of the pericardial, pleural, and peritoneal cavities; kidneys and ureters

   C. Umbilical cord
      1. The cord serves as the lifeline from the EMBRYO to the placenta
      2. It measures from 20″ to 22″ (50 to 55 cm) in length and ¾″ (2 cm) in diameter at term
      3. The cord contains two arteries and one vein
      4. It also contains Wharton's jelly, a gelatinous substance that helps prevent kinking of the cord in utero
      5. Blood flows through the cord at about 400 ml/minute

   D. Placenta
      1. The placenta contains 15 to 20 subdivisions called COTYLEDONS
      2. The placenta weighs approximately 1 to 1.3 lb (450 to 600 g), measures from 6″ to 10″ (15 to 25 cm) in diameter, and is 1″ to 1¼″ (2.5 to 3 cm) thick at term
      3. Having a rough texture, the placenta appears red on the maternal surface and shiny and gray on the fetal surface
      4. The placenta functions as a transport mechanism between the mother and the FETUS
         a. The placenta's life span and function depend on oxygen consumption and maternal circulation; circulation to the fetus and placenta improves when the mother lies on her left side
         b. The placenta receives maternal oxygen via diffusion

      c. It produces hormones, including human chorionic gonadotropin, human placental lactogen, gonadotropin-releasing hormone, thyrotropin-releasing factor, corticotropin, estrogen, and progesterone

      d. It supplies the fetus with carbohydrates, water, fats, protein, minerals, and inorganic salts

      e. It carries end products of fetal metabolism to the maternal circulation for excretion

      f. It transfers passive immunity via maternal antibodies

E. Amniotic fluid

  1. At term, the uterus contains 800 to 1,200 ml of amniotic fluid, which is clear and yellowish and has a specific gravity of 1.007 to 1.025 and a pH of 7.0 to 7.25

  2. Maternal serum provides amniotic fluid in early gestation, with increasing amounts derived from fetal urine late in gestation

  3. Amniotic fluid is replaced every 3 hours

  4. Contents include albumin, lanugo, urea, creatinine, bilirubin, fat, enzymes, lecithin, sphingomyelin, and leukocytes

  5. Amniotic fluid prevents heat loss, preserves constant fetal body temperatures, cushions the fetus, and facilitates fetal growth and development

F. Fetal circulation structures (see also *Fetal blood circulation,* page 18)

  1. *Umbilical vein* carries oxygenated blood to the fetus from the placenta

  2. *Umbilical arteries* carry deoxygenated blood from the fetus to the placenta

  3. *Foramen ovale* serves as the septal opening between the atria of the fetal heart

  4. *Ductus arteriosus* connects the pulmonary artery to the aorta, allowing blood to shunt around the fetal lungs

  5. *Ductus venosus* carries oxygenated blood from the umbilical vein to the inferior vena cava, bypassing the liver

G. Gestational age development

  1. As the embryo grows, different patterns and structures develop

  2. By the 4th week of gestation, a normal fetus begins to show noticeable signs of growth in all areas assessed (see *Fetal development by gestational age,* pages 19 to 22)

CLINICAL ALERT

  3. Failure to feel fetal movement after the 20th week of gestation must be investigated by the health care provider

Text continues on page 22.

Fetal blood circulation

The three flow charts below illustrate fetal blood circulation. The first chart shows the flow of blood from the placenta to the inferior vena cava. After the blood reaches the inferior vena cava, most of the blood flows back to the placenta, as shown in the second chart. However, a small amount of blood flows differently, taking the path shown in the third chart.

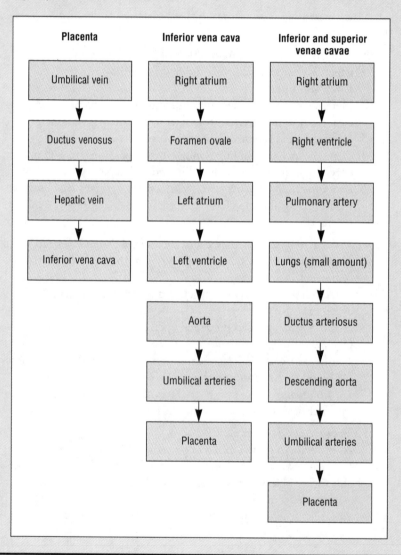

Placenta	**Inferior vena cava**	**Inferior and superior venae cavae**
Umbilical vein	Right atrium	Right atrium
Ductus venosus	Foramen ovale	Right ventricle
Hepatic vein	Left atrium	Pulmonary artery
Inferior vena cava	Left ventricle	Lungs (small amount)
	Aorta	Ductus arteriosus
	Umbilical arteries	Descending aorta
	Placenta	Umbilical arteries
		Placenta

Fetal development by gestational age

This chart highlights significant areas of fetal growth and development by body system, along with changes in appearance and weight and crown-to-rump measurements. Weeks are approximate.

BODY SYSTEM	GESTATIONAL AGE (in weeks)	DEVELOPMENT
Respiratory	4 to 7	Primary lung, tracheal, and bronchi buds appear. Nasal pits form. Abdominal and thoracic cavities are separated by the diaphragm.
	8 to 12	Bronchioles branch. Pleural and pericardial cavities appear. Lungs assume definitive shape.
	13 to 20	Terminal and respiratory bronchioles appear.
	21 to 28	Nostrils open. Surfactant production begins. Respiratory movements are possible. Alveolar ducts and sacs appear.
	38 to 40	Pulmonary branching is two-thirds complete. Lecithin-sphingomyelin ratio is 2:1.
Genitourinary	4 to 7	Rudimentary ureteral buds are present.
	8 to 12	Bladder and urethra separate from rectum; bladder expands as a sac. Kidneys secrete urine.
	13 to 20	Kidneys are in proper position with definitive shape.
	36	Nephron formation ceases.
Nervous	4	Midbrain flexure is well-marked.
	8	Cerebral cortex, meninges, ventricular foramens, and cerebrospinal fluid circulation are differentiated.
	12 to 16	Brain structural configuration is roughly completed. Cerebral lobes are delineated. Cerebellum assumes prominence.
	20 to 24	Brain is grossly formed. Myelination of spinal cord begins. Spinal cord ends at S-1.
	28 to 36	Cerebral fissures and convolutions appear. Spinal cord ends at L-3.
	40	Myelination of brain begins. *(continued)*

Fetal development by gestational age (continued)

BODY SYSTEM	GESTATIONAL AGE (in weeks)	DEVELOPMENT
Gastrointestinal	4	Oral cavity and primitive jaw are present. Stomach, ducts of pancreas, and liver form. Esophagus and trachea division begins.
	8 to 11	Intestinal villi form. Small intestines coil in umbilical cord.
	12 to 16	Bile is secreted. Intestines withdraw from umbilical cord to normal position. Meconium is present in bowel. Anus opens.
	20	Enamel and dentin are deposited. Ascending colon appears. Fetus can suck and swallow. Peristaltic movements begin.
Hepatic	4	Liver function begins.
	6	Liver hematopoiesis begins.
Endocrine	2 to 3	Thyroid tissue appears.
	4	Thyroid can synthesize thyroxine.
	10	Islets of Langerhans differentiated.
	12	Thyroid secretes hormones. Insulin present in pancreas.
Reproductive	2 to 3	Sex is determined.
	6 to 8	Sex glands appear and begin differentiation into ovaries or testes. External genitalia appear similar.
	12 to 24	Testes descend into the inguinal canal. External genitalia are distinguishable.
Musculoskeletal	4	Limb buds appear.
	8	Ossification (mandible, humerus, occiput) is identifiable.
	12	Some bones are well outlined. Ossification continues.
	16	Joint cavities are present. Muscular movements are detectable.
	20	Ossification of sternum is identifiable. Mother can detect fetal movements (quickening).

Fetal development by gestational age (continued)

BODY SYSTEM	GESTATIONAL AGE (in weeks)	DEVELOPMENT
Musculoskeletal (continued)	28 to 32	Ossification continues. Fetus can turn head to side.
	36	Muscle tone is developed; fetus can turn and elevate head.
Cardiovascular	2 to 4	Heart formation begins. Blood circulation begins. Primitive RBCs circulate. Fetus has tubular heartbeat by 24 days.
	5 to 7	Atria divide. Heart chambers are present. Fetal heartbeat is detectable. Blood cell groups are identifiable.
	8	Heart development is complete. Fetal circulation follows two intraembryonic and four extraembryonic circuits.
	12 to 20	Fetal heart tones are audible with Doppler (12 weeks) and fetoscope (16 to 20).
External appearance	4	Body is C-shaped; eyes pigmented; auditory pit enclosed.
	8	Eyes, ears, nose, and mouth recognizable; flat nose; eyes far apart; digits well formed.
	12	Nails appear; skin is pink and delicate; lacrimal ducts developing.
	16	Head is dominant; scalp hair present; sweat glands developing.
	20	Vernix, lanugo, and sebaceous glands appear; legs considerably lengthened.
	24	Skin red and wrinkled; eyes structurally complete.
	28	Eyelids open.
	32	Subcutaneous fat increases; skin pink and smooth.
	36	Lanugo disappearing; earlobes soft with little cartilage.
	40	Vernix is copious; hair is moderate to profuse; lanugo on shoulders and upper body; ear lobes stiffer with cartilage. *(continued)*

Fetal development by gestational age (continued)

GESTATIONAL AGE (in weeks)	WEIGHT (g)	CROWN-TO-RUMP LENGTH (cm)
4	0.4	0.4 to 0.5
8	2	2.5 to 3.0
12	19	6.0 to 9.0
16	100	11.5 to 13.5
20	300	16.0 to 18.5
24	600	23
28	1,100	27
32	1,800 to 2,100	31
36	2,200 to 2,900	35
40	3,200+	40

POINTS TO REMEMBER

◆ All embryonic tissues and organs are derived from the ectoderm, the endoderm, or the mesoderm.

◆ The umbilical cord is the fetus's lifeline to its mother.

◆ Embryonic maturation follows distinct patterns, although exact timing of development may differ.

STUDY QUESTIONS

To evaluate your understanding of this chapter, answer the following questions in the space provided; then compare your responses with the correct answers in Appendix B, page 172.

1. Where are the male and female gametes produced? _____

   _____

   _____

2. When does the morula change into a blastocyst? _____

   _____

   _____

3. What is the endometrium called after implantation of the blastocyst? _____

   _____

   _____

4. What are the two fetal membranes?_____

   _____

   _____

5. On what does placental function depend? _____

   _____

   _____

CRITICAL THINKING AND APPLICATION EXERCISES

1. Research the process of mitosis and meiosis. Develop a chart comparing and contrasting the events of each phase.

2. Create a table identifying the hormones produced by the placenta and the functions and effects of each.

3. Compare and contrast fetal circulation with extrauterine circulation.

CHAPTER

The Normal Prenatal Period

LEARNING OBJECTIVES

After studying this chapter, you should be able to:

♦ Describe the physiologic and psychological adaptations to pregnancy.

♦ Explain causes of and interventions for common discomforts of pregnancy.

♦ Describe common methods for assessing fetal status.

♦ Identify major points to include when counseling a pregnant patient.

♦ Describe the nutritional needs of the pregnant patient.

CHAPTER OVERVIEW

A woman who is pregnant experiences presumptive, probable, and positive signs of pregnancy. Pregnancy causes normal physiologic changes in each body system and psychosocial adaptations. Many of the discomforts of pregnancy are related to these physiologic changes. Nursing care during the normal prenatal period involves obtaining a thorough maternal history and physical examination, and patient education about health promotion activities, nutrition, and danger signs to be reported.

◆ I. Signs and symptoms of pregnancy

A. Presumptive
   1. Amenorrhea (in about 80% of patients) or slight, painless spotting of unknown cause in early gestation (in about 20% of patients)
   2. Nausea and vomiting
   3. Urinary frequency and urgency
   4. Breast enlargement and tenderness
   5. Fatigue
   6. Quickening
   7. Thinning and softening of fingernails
   8. Intensified skin pigmentation

B. Probable
   1. Uterine enlargement
   2. Goodell's sign (softening of the cervix)
   3. Chadwick's sign (bluish mucous membranes of the vagina, cervix, and vulva)
   4. Hegar's sign (softening of the lower uterine segment)
   5. Braxton Hicks contractions (painless uterine contractions that recur throughout pregnancy)
   6. Ballottement (passive fetal movement in response to tapping of the lower portion of the uterus or cervix)
   7. Positive pregnancy test results

C. Positive
   1. Fetal heartbeat detected by 17 to 20 weeks of gestation
   2. Ultrasonography results as early as 6 weeks of gestation
   3. Fetal movements felt by examiner after 16 weeks of gestation

◆ II. Physiologic adaptations to pregnancy

A. Cardiovascular system
   1. Cardiac hypertrophy from increased blood volume and cardiac output
   2. Displacement of the heart upward and to the left from pressure on the diaphragm
   3. Progressive increase in blood volume, peaking in the third trimester at 30% to 50% of prepregnancy levels
   4. Resting pulse rate fluctuations, with increases ranging from 0 to 15 beats/minute at term
   5. Pulmonic systolic and apical systolic murmurs resulting from decreased blood viscosity and increased blood flow
   6. Increased femoral venous pressure caused by impaired circulation from the lower extremities (this results from the pressure of the enlarged uterus on the pelvic veins and inferior vena cava)

    7. Decreased cerebrospinal fluid space from enlargement of vessels surrounding the spinal cord's dura mater

    8. Increased fibrinogen levels (up to 50% at term) from hormonal influences

    9. Increased levels of blood coagulation factors VII, IX, and X, leading to a hypercoagulable state

    10. Increase of about 33% in total red blood cell volume, despite hemodilution and decreasing erythrocyte count

    11. Hematocrit decrease of approximately 7%

    12. Total hemoglobin increase of 12% to 15%; this is less than the overall plasma volume increase, thus reducing hemoglobin concentration and leading to physiologic anemia of pregnancy

    13. Leukocyte production equal to or slightly greater than blood volume increase (average leukocyte count is 10,000 to 11,000/µl; this peaks at 25,000/µl during labor, possibly through an estrogen-related mechanism)

B. Gastrointestinal system

    1. Gum swelling from increased estrogen levels; gums may be spongy and hyperemic

    2. Lateral and posterior displacement of the intestines

    3. Superior and lateral displacement of the stomach

    4. Delayed intestinal motility and gastric and gallbladder emptying time from smooth muscle relaxation caused by high levels of placental progesterone

    5. Hemorrhoids in late pregnancy from venous pressure

    6. Constipation from increased progesterone levels, resulting in increased water absorption from the colon

    7. Displacement of the appendix from McBurney's point (making diagnosis of appendicitis difficult)

C. Endocrine system

    1. Increased basal metabolic rate (up 25% at term) caused by demands of the fetus and uterus and by increased oxygen consumption

    2. Increased iodine metabolism from slight hyperplasia of the thyroid caused by estrogen levels

    3. Slight parathyroidism from increased requirement for calcium and vitamin D

    4. Elevated plasma parathyroid hormone levels, peaking between 15 and 35 weeks of gestation

    5. Slightly enlarged pituitary gland

    6. Increased production of prolactin by the pituitary gland

    7. Increased estrogen levels and hypertrophy of the adrenal cortex

    8. Increased cortisol levels to regulate protein and carbohydrate metabolism

    9. Decreased maternal blood glucose levels

  10. Decreased insulin production in early pregnancy

  11. Increased production of estrogen, progesterone, and human chorionic somatomammotropin by the placenta, and increased levels of maternal cortisol, which reduce the mother's ability to use insulin, thus ensuring an adequate glucose supply for the fetus and placenta

D. Respiratory system

    1. Increased vascularization of the respiratory tract caused by estrogen levels

    2. Shortening of the lungs caused by the enlarging uterus

    3. Upward displacement of the diaphragm by the uterus

    4. Increased tidal volume, causing slight hyperventilation

    5. Increased chest circumference (by approximately $2\frac{3}{8}''$ [5.5 cm])

    6. Altered breathing, with abdominal breathing replacing thoracic breathing as pregnancy progresses

    7. Slight increase (2 breaths/minute) in respiratory rate

    8. Lowered threshold for carbon dioxide from estrogen and progesterone

E. Metabolic system

    1. Increased water retention caused by higher levels of steroidal sex hormones, decreased serum protein levels, and increased intracapillary pressure and permeability

    2. Increased levels of serum lipids, lipoproteins, and cholesterol

    3. Increased iron requirements caused by fetal demands

    4. Increased carbohydrate needs

    5. Increased protein retention from hyperplasia and hypertrophy of maternal tissues

    6. Weight gain of 25 to 30 lb (11.3 to 13.6 kg)

      a. Commonly estimated at 3-, 12-, and 12-lb (1.4-, 5.4-, 5.4-kg) gains for first, second, and third trimesters, respectively

      b. Caused by fetus (7.5 lb [3.4 kg]), placenta and membranes (1.5 lb [0.7 kg]), amniotic fluid (2 lb [0.9 kg]), uterus (2.5 lb [1.1 kg]), breasts (3 lb [1.4 kg]), blood volume (2 to 4 lb [0.9 to 1.8 kg]), and extravascular fluid and fat reserves (4 to 9 lb [1.8 to 4.1 kg])

F. Integumentary system

    1. Hyperactive sweat and sebaceous glands

    2. Changing pigmentation from the increase of melanocyte-stimulating hormone caused by increased estrogen and progesterone levels

      a. Nipples, areola, cervix, vagina, and vulva darken

      b. Nose, cheeks, and forehead show pigmentary changes known as facial chloasma

G. Genitourinary system
   1. Dilated ureters and renal pelvis caused by progesterone and pressure from the enlarging uterus
   2. Increased glomerular filtration rate (GFR) and renal plasma flow (RPF) early in pregnancy; GFR is elevated until delivery, whereas RPF returns to a near-normal level by term
   3. Increased clearance of urea and creatinine from increased renal function
   4. Decreased blood urea and nonprotein nitrogen values from increased renal function
   5. Glucosuria from increased glomerular filtration without an increase in tubular reabsorptive capacity
   6. Decreased bladder tone
   7. Increased sodium retention from hormonal influences
   8. Increases in dimensions of uterus
      a. From approximately 2½″ to 12½″ (6.5 to 32 cm) in length
      b. From 1½″ to 9½″ (4 to 24 cm) in width
      c. From 8⅝″ to 10″ (22 to 25 cm) in depth
      d. From approximately 2 to 42 oz (55 to 1,200 g) in weight
      e. From approximately ⅛ to 170 oz (3.5 ml to 5,000 ml) in volume
   9. Hypertrophied uterine muscle cells (5 to 10 times normal size)
   10. Increased vascularity, edema, hypertrophy, and hyperplasia of the cervical glands
   11. Increased vaginal secretions with a pH of 3.5 to 6
   12. Discontinued ovulation and maturation of new follicles
   13. Thickening of vaginal mucosa, loosening of vaginal connective tissue, and hypertrophy of small muscle cells

◆ III. Psychological adaptations to pregnancy

A. General information
   1. Psychological responses to pregnancy may vary because of hormonal changes, altered body image, anticipation of role changes, emotional makeup and sociocultural background, and reactions of family and friends
   2. Common responses include ambivalence, acceptance, introversion, and emotional lability
   3. Unresolved emotional conflicts between the patient and her mother, fear of pending role changes or of labor and delivery, and the need to alter career plans can cause mixed feelings, even when the pregnancy was planned

4. As the pregnancy progresses, the patient's changing physical appearance, quickening, and hearing fetal heart tones usually help her accept the pregnancy and perceive the fetus as real

5. The patient may turn her attention toward herself to prepare for the birth; although this is normal, it may strain the relationship if her partner misinterprets introversion as rejection

6. Wide mood swings can strain marital or familial relationships, possibly causing the partner or family members to withdraw, leaving the patient feeling rejected

B. Developmental tasks

1. Depending on the woman's age, developmental tasks during pregnancy may include acceptance and comfort with body image, development of a personal value system, adjustment to an adult identity, and internalization of sexual role and identity

2. Tasks of pregnancy include acceptance of the pregnancy, the pregnancy's termination at the time of delivery, and the maternal role; and resolution of fears regarding childbirth and bonding

♦ IV. Common discomforts during the first trimester

A. Nausea and vomiting ("morning sickness," but symptoms may occur at any time)

1. Causes: hormonal changes, fatigue, emotional factors, and changes in carbohydrate metabolism

2. Patient teaching: avoid greasy, highly seasoned food; eat small, frequent meals; eat dry toast or crackers before arising in the morning

B. Nasal stuffiness, discharge, or obstruction

1. Cause: edema of the nasal mucosa from elevated estrogen levels

2. Patient teaching: use a cool-air vaporizer

C. Breast enlargement and tenderness

1. Cause: increased estrogen and progesterone levels

2. Patient teaching: wear a well-fitting bra

D. Urinary frequency and urgency

1. Cause: pressure of the enlarging uterus on the bladder (around the 12th week, the uterus rises into the abdominal cavity, causing symptoms to disappear; they recur in the third trimester as the uterus again presses on the bladder)

2. Patient teaching: decrease fluid intake in the evening to minimize nocturia; limit caffeine-containing fluids; respond to the urge to void immediately to prevent bladder distention and urine stasis; perform Kegel exercises; promptly report signs of urinary tract infection

E. Increased LEUKORRHEA

1. Causes: hyperplasia of vaginal mucosa, increased mucus production by the endocervical glands
2. Patient teaching: bathe daily and wear absorbent cotton underwear

◆ V. Common discomforts during the second and third trimesters

A. Heartburn

1. Causes: relaxation of the cardiac sphincter, decreased gastrointestinal motility, increased production of progesterone, gastric displacement
2. Patient teaching: eat small, frequent meals; avoid fatty or fried foods; remain upright for at least 1 hour after eating; use antacids that do not contain sodium bicarbonate

B. Constipation

1. Causes: oral iron supplements, displacement of the intestines by the fetus, bowel sluggishness caused by increased progesterone and steroid metabolism
2. Patient teaching: exercise daily, increase fluid intake and dietary bulk, maintain regular elimination patterns

C. Hemorrhoids

1. Cause: pressure on the pelvic veins by the enlarging uterus, which interferes with venous circulation
2. Patient teaching: avoid constipation, prolonged standing, and constrictive clothing; use topical ointments, warm soaks, and anesthetic agents

D. Backache

1. Cause: postural adjustments of pregnancy (curvature of the lumbosacral vertebrae increases as the uterus enlarges)
2. Patient teaching: use proper body mechanics, maintain good posture, avoid high heels

E. Leg cramps

1. Causes: pressure from the enlarging uterus, poor circulation, fatigue, and an imbalance in the calcium-phosphorus ratio
2. Patient teaching: alter calcium and phosphorus intake, frequently rest with legs raised, wear warm clothing; during a leg cramp, pull the toes up toward the leg while pressing down on the knee

F. Shortness of breath

1. Cause: pressure of the uterus on the diaphragm
2. Patient teaching: maintain proper posture, especially when standing; use semi-Fowler's position when sleeping

G. Ankle edema
   1. Causes: poor venous return from the lower extremities; aggravated by prolonged sitting or standing and by warm weather
   2. Patient teaching: avoid tight garments; elevate the legs during rest periods, and ensure dorsiflexion of the feet if standing or sitting for prolonged periods

♦ **VI. Estimated date of delivery and gestational age assessments**

A. Nägele's rule
   1. Nägele's rule determines the estimated date of delivery
   2. The procedure is as follows:
      a. Subtract 3 months from the first day of the last menstrual period
      b. Add 7 days (for example, October 5 - 3 months = July 5 + 7 days = July 12)

B. Fetal movement
   1. Fetal movement, also called quickening, is described as a light fluttering
   2. It usually is felt first between 16 and 22 weeks of gestation

C. Fetal heart sounds
   1. Fetal heart sounds can be detected at 12 weeks of gestation with a Doppler ultrasound.
   2. They also can be auscultated at 16 to 20 weeks with a fetoscope

D. Fetal crown-to-rump measurements
   1. Fetal crown-to-rump measurements are determined by ultrasonography
   2. They can be used to assess the fetus's age until the head can be defined

E. Biparietal diameter
   1. Biparietal diameter is the widest transverse diameter of the fetal head.
   2. Measurements can be made by about 12 to 13 weeks of gestation

F. Fundal height
   1. Fundal height is difficult to interpret
   2. The measurement can be affected by the patient's weight, polyhydramnios, more than one fetus (multiple gestation), and the fetus's size
   3. McDonald's rule uses fundal height to determine the duration of a pregnancy in either lunar months or weeks
   4. To use this rule, place a tape measure at the symphysis pubis and measure up and over the fundus. Fundal height in cm $\times \frac{2}{7}$ = duration of pregnancy in lunar months; fundal height in cm $\times \frac{8}{7}$ = duration of pregnancy in weeks

◆ VII. Monitoring fetal status

A. Amniocentesis (insertion of a spinal needle into the uterus transabdominally to aspirate amniotic fluid for analysis)
1. Performed after the 14th week of gestation, when amniotic fluid is sufficient and the uterus has moved into the abdominal cavity
2. Preceded by ultrasound to locate the fetus, placenta, and fluid
3. Followed by at least 30 minutes of monitoring fetal heart rate and uterine activity with an external fetal monitor

CLINICAL ALERT

4. Carries the risk of maternal hemorrhage, infection, premature labor, fetal hemorrhage, and amnionitis
5. Used for assessment, diagnosis, and evaluation
   a. Prenatal diagnosis of genetic disorders, such as chromosomal aberrations, sex-linked disorders, inborn errors of metabolism, and neural tube defects

CLINICAL ALERT

   b. Diagnosis and evaluation of isoimmune disease, including Rh sensitization and ABO incompatibility; Rh negative mothers must receive Rhogam following amniocentesis
   c. Gestational age assessment via a LECITHIN-SPHINGOMYELIN ratio, presence of phosphatidyl glycerol, creatinine levels, or the delta optical density of bilirubinoid pigments

B. Chorionic villi sampling (CVS) (removal and analysis of a small tissue specimen from the fetal portion of the placenta to determine the genetic makeup of the fetus)
1. CVS sampling provides an earlier diagnosis, allows an earlier and safer abortion if chosen, and produces less social and psychological stress than amniocentesis because results are received earlier in gestation (can be performed as early as the eighth week)

CLINICAL ALERT

2. It carries the risk of spontaneous abortion, infection, hematoma, and intrauterine death
3. Rh negative mother must receive Rhogam following CVS

C. Ultrasonography (ultrasound waves reflected by tissues of different densities; signals are amplified and displayed on an oscilloscope or screen)
1. Is noninvasive and painless
2. Provides immediate results without potential harm to the fetus or the mother
3. Can detect fetal death, malformation, malpresentations, placental abnormalities, multiple gestation, and hydramnios or oligohydramnios

D. Fetal movement
   1. Can be identified by the patient 90% of the time
   2. Is affected by drugs, cigarettes, sound, time of day, sleep patterns, and blood glucose levels
   3. Indicates fetal well-being (at least two movements per hour)

E. Non-stress test (NST; noninvasive test to detect fetal heart accelerations either spontaneously or in response to fetal movement)
   1. Provides immediate results simply and inexpensively without contraindications or complications
   2. Benefits a patient at risk for uteroplacental insufficiency and altered fetal movements
   3. Can be begun between 32 and 34 weeks of gestation
   4. Indicates the possibility of fetal hypoxia, fetal sleep cycle, or the effects of drugs when nonreactive (see *Interpreting NST and OCT results,* page 34)

F. Stress test (oxytocin challenge test [OCT]; method of evaluating fetal ability to withstand the physiologic stress of an oxytocin-induced contraction)
   1. Involves I.V. administration of oxytocin, usually starting at 0.5 mU/minute and increasing by 0.5 mU/minute at 15- to 20-minute intervals until three high-quality uterine contractions are obtained within 10 minutes
   2. Used with a patient at risk for placental insufficiency or fetal compromise from diabetes, heart disease, hypertension, history of previous stillbirth, renal disease, or a nonreactive NST
   3. Does not apply to those with previous classical cesarean section, third trimester bleeding, or high risk for preterm labor
   4. Can be begun at 32 to 34 weeks of gestation
   5. Requires fetal heart rate pattern evaluation for early, late, and variable decelerations

G. Nipple stimulation stress test (breast self-stimulation test)
   1. Induces contractions by activating sensory receptors in the areola, triggering the release of oxytocin by the posterior pituitary gland
   2. May require nipple-rolling or applying warm washcloths to one nipple
   3. Is noninvasive, less expensive, and less time-consuming than the OCT but carries the risk of hyperstimulation or embarrassment
   4. Has the same reactive pattern as the reactive NST result
   5. Has the same positive pattern as the positive OCT result

H. Vibroacoustic stimulation (uses vibration and sound to induce fetal reactivity during an NST)
   1. Is noninvasive and convenient; NST results are quickly obtained
   2. Uses an artificial larynx or fetal acoustic stimulator to apply stimulation for 1 to 5 seconds over the fetus's head

Interpreting NST and OCT results

The following chart lists the possible interpretations of results from a nonstress test (NST) and an oxytocin challenge test (OCT), commonly called a stress test. Appropriate actions are also included.

NST RESULT	INTERPRETATION	ACTION
Reactive	Two or more fetal heart rate accelerations of 15 beats/minute lasting 15 seconds or more within 20 minutes	Repeat NST bi-weekly or weekly, depending on rationale for testing.
Nonreactive	Tracing without fetal heart rate (FHR) accelerations or with accelerations of fewer than 15 beats/minute lasting less than 15 seconds throughout fetal movement	Repeat in 24 hours or perform a biophysical profile immediately.
Unsatisfactory	Quality of FHR recording inadequate for interpretation	Repeat in 24 hours or perform a biophysical profile immediately.
OCT RESULT	**INTERPRETATION**	**ACTION**
Negative	No late decelerations; three contractions every 10 minutes; fetus would probably survive labor if it occurred within 1 week	No further action needed now.
Positive	Persistent and consistent late decelerations with more than half of contractions	Induce labor; fetus is at risk for perinatal morbidity and mortality.
Suspicious	Late decelerations with less than half of contractions after an adequate contraction pattern has been established	Repeat test in 24 hours.
Hyperstimulation	Late decelerations with excessive uterine activity (occurring more often than every 2 minutes or lasting longer than 90 seconds)	Repeat test in 24 hours.
Unsatisfactory	Poor monitor tracing or uterine contraction pattern	Repeat test in 24 hours.

I. Biophysical profile
   1. Assesses five biophysical variables: fetal breathing movements, body movements, muscle tone, amniotic fluid volume, and fetal heart rate reactivity
   2. Is noninvasive and relatively quick to perform
   3. Can detect central nervous system depression

J. Fetal blood flow studies
   1. Umbilical or uterine doppler velocimetry aids in evaluating fetal status, especially in patients with hypertension, diabetes, isoimmunization and lupus
   2. It is indicated in the fetus with suspected congenital anomalies or cardiac arrhythmias

K. Percutaneous umbilical blood sampling (PUBS)
   1. PUBS is an invasive procedure during which a spinal needle is inserted into the umbilical cord, under direct ultrasound guidance
   2. Procedure is performed to obtain fetal blood samples or to transfuse the fetus in utero
   3. It is used when fetus is at risk for congenital and chromosomal abnormalities, congenital infection, or anemia

   4. Rh-negative mothers must receive RhoGAM following PUBS

◆ **VIII. Maternal assessment**

A. Maternal physical examination
   1. Breasts
      a. Inspection
      b. Palpation
   2. Abdomen
      a. Inspection
      b. Auscultation
      c. Percussion
      d. Palpation
   3. External genitalia
      a. Inspection of pubic hair, skin, labia, clitoris, urethral orifice, perineum, and anus
      b. Palpation of the mons pubis, inguinal lymphatics, labia, and Skene's and Bartholin's glands
   4. Speculum examination
      a. Cervix
      b. Papanicolaou's smear
      c. Vaginal mucosa
   5. Bimanual abdominovaginal palpation
      a. Cervix
      b. Uterus

      c. CUL-DE-SAC

      d. ADNEXAL AREA

    6. Rectovaginal palpation

      a. Uterus

      b. Adnexal area

      c. Cul-de-sac

    7. Smears for cytology

      a. Cervical

      b. Endocervical

      c. Vaginal

B. Maternal medical and obstetric history

    1. Past medical history

      a. Childhood diseases

      b. Surgical procedures

      c. Medical problems (such as hypertension, renal, or cardiac disease)

    2. Family medical history

      a. History of multiple births, congenital diseases, or deformities

      b. Significant medical problems

    3. Present medical status

      a. Prescription and nonprescription medications

      b. Use of alcohol, tobacco, or illegal drugs

      c. Conditions that could negatively affect pregnancy (for example, viral infection)

      d. Presence of disease, such as diabetes or cardiac disease

    4. Obstetric history

      a. Number of pregnancies, abortions (spontaneous and induced), and living children; list total number of pregnancies, number of premature deliveries, number of abortions and miscarriages, number of living children

      b. History of previous pregnancies (antepartum, intrapartum, and postpartum)

      c. Perinatal status of previous neonates

    5. Current pregnancy

      a. First day of last menstrual period

      b. Abnormal symptoms (cramping, vaginal bleeding)

      c. Attitude toward pregnancy

    6. Gynecologic history

      a. History of infections (cervical, vaginal, or sexually transmitted)

      b. Age at menarche; typical menstrual-cycle characteristics

      c. Contraceptive use

    7. Partner's history

      a. Age

      b. Genetic or medical disorders

      c. Alcohol or drug use

8. Personal information
   a. Age, religion, economic status, and educational level
   b. History of emotional or psychiatric disorders
   c. Diet practices

C. Routine maternal laboratory testing
   1. Rubella titer to assess immunity to rubella
   2. Complete blood count to detect anemia or infection
   3. Blood type, Rh, and abnormal antibodies to identify the fetus at risk for erythroblastosis fetalis or hyperbilirubinemia
   4. Rapid plasma reagin to detect untreated syphilis
   5. Serum glucose to detect gestational diabetes
   6. Urinalysis and urine culture to test for glucose, protein, blood, acetone, and asymptomatic bacteriuria
   7. Hepatitis B to screen for presence of Hepatitis B surface antigen
   8. Gonorrhea smear and chlamydia to detect sexually transmitted diseases
   9. Triple screen between 15-20 weeks to identify fetus at increased risk for Down syndrome and neural tube defects

♦ IX. Patient counseling

A. Childbirth and parenthood education
   1. Classes address the learning needs of the parents-to-be
   2. Topics include nutrition, labor and delivery, breathing exercises, and anesthesia and analgesia

B. Dental care
   1. A dental checkup early in pregnancy is encouraged
   2. Nausea and vomiting, heartburn, and hyperemia of gums may lead to poor oral hygiene and dental caries
   3. The fetus receives calcium and phosphorus from the pregnant patient's diet, not from her teeth; the belief that a patient loses a tooth for every pregnancy is a fallacy

C. Immunizations
   1. Immunizations with attenuated live viruses (including mumps and rubella vaccines) should not be given during pregnancy because of their teratogenic effect on the developing embryo
   2. Vaccinations with killed viruses (including varicella, hepatitis, influenza, tetanus, and diphtheria vaccines) may be given during pregnancy

D. Clothing
   1. Clothes should be nonconstrictive
   2. Low-heeled shoes help prevent backache and poor balance

3. Maternity girdles are rarely needed; however, a patient with a pendulous abdomen may benefit from decreased curvature of the spine

E. Danger signs to report immediately
   1. Severe vomiting
   2. Frequent and severe headaches
   3. Epigastric pain
   4. Fluid discharge from vagina
   5. Fetal movement changes or cessation after quickening
   6. Swelling of the fingers or face
   7. Visual disturbances
   8. Signs of vaginal or urinary tract infection
   9. Unusual or severe abdominal pain
   10. Seizures or muscular irritability

F. Substance abuse
   1. Abuse increases risk of gross structural fetal defects (greatest in the first trimester, during organogenesis)
   2. Smoking
      a. Causes vasoconstriction
      b. Alters maternal and fetal heart rate
      c. Alters blood pressure and cardiac output
      d. Increases the incidence of low-birth-weight infants
   3. Alcohol and drugs affect the fetus and neonate

G. Medications: a pregnant patient should consult a doctor before taking any medication

H. Sexuality
   1. Sexual behavior (coital and noncoital) is usually unrestricted in complication-free pregnancies
   2. Sexual desire may decrease during the first trimester from discomforts and fatigue
   3. Sexual desire may increase in the second trimester, when discomforts commonly wane; the woman may have greater sexual satisfaction than before pregnancy because of vascular congestion of the pelvis
   4. Sexual desire may decrease in the third trimester from increasing fatigue and abdominal size

I. Physical activities and precautions
   1. Prenatal exercises increase muscle strength in preparation for delivery and promote restoration of muscle tone after delivery
   2. Kegel exercises strengthen the pubococcygeal muscle and increase its elasticity

TEACHING TIPS
Pregnant patient during the prenatal period

Be sure to include the following topics in your teaching plan for the pregnant patient during the prenatal period:
- Physiologic changes and psychosocial adaptations
- Possible diagnostic procedures
- Common discomforts
- Danger signs
- Self-care and health promotion activities
- Avoidance of medication use
- Nutritional requirements and appropriate food choices

      3. The work site should be checked for potential environmental hazards, such as pesticides, anesthetic gas, and such heavy metals as lead and mercury
      4. Obstetric complications may deter employment during pregnancy
      5. Work duties may have to be altered to avoid excessive physical strain
      6. Seat belts should be worn low, under the abdomen

J. Breast care
      1. Proper breast support promotes comfort, retains breast shape, and prevents back strain
      2. For additional teaching tips, see *Pregnant patient during the prenatal period*

♦ X. Nutrition during pregnancy

A. Calories
      1. Requirement during pregnancy exceeds prepregnancy needs by 300 calories/day (from 2,100 kcal/day to 2,400 kcal/day)
      2. Extra calories are needed to:
         a. Support maternal-fetal tissue synthesis
         b. Meet increased basal metabolic needs
         c. Provide optimal use of protein and tissue growth

B. Protein
      1. Requirement during pregnancy exceeds prepregnancy needs by 30 g/day (from 46 g/day to 76 g/day)
      2. Increased protein intake is needed for:
         a. Expansion of blood volume
         b. Tissue growth
         c. Provision of adequate amino acids for fetal development

C. Vitamins
      1. Intake of all vitamins should be increased

2. Increase is needed for tissue synthesis and energy production
3. Folic acid is particularly important
    a. It promotes fetal growth and prevents anemia
    b. Intake should be increased from 400 mg/day to 800 mg/day
    c. Sources of folic acid include green, leafy vegetables; eggs; milk; and whole-grain breads

D. Minerals
1. Intake of all minerals, especially iron, should be increased
2. The average American diet does not provide enough iron to prevent iron-deficiency anemia; recommended supplemental iron intake is 30 to 60 mg/day

CLINICAL ALERT

3. Sodium restriction is no longer advocated because it has been associated with hormonal and biochemical changes.
    a. The National Research Council recommends an increase in daily sodium intake of 69 mg over the normal dietary requirement of 2,400 mg
    b. Excessive sodium may lead to hypertension by altering fluid and electrolyte balance

POINTS TO REMEMBER

♦ Comprehensive prenatal care is essential for the health of the pregnant patient and her fetus.

♦ A thorough maternal physical examination and history increases the chances of a successful pregnancy.

♦ Pregnancy may represent a developmental crisis for the patient and her family.

♦ The nurse must understand the normal physical and psychological changes of pregnancy to identify deviations from normal.

STUDY QUESTIONS

To evaluate your understanding of this chapter, answer the following questions in the space provided; then compare your responses with the correct answers in Appendix B, pages 172 and 173.

1. What are the probable signs of pregnancy? _____
_____
_____

2. During pregnancy, what happens to the heart from displacement of the diaphragm? _____

_____

_____

3. What are the common psychological responses to pregnancy? _____

_____

_____

4. How can the nurse intervene for a patient with breast enlargement and tenderness in the first trimester? _____

_____

_____

5. What are common discomforts of the second and third trimesters? _____

_____

_____

6. How is the estimated date of delivery determined using Nägele's rule? _____

_____

_____

7. What does a reactive NST indicate? _____

_____

_____

8. Which five variables are evaluated on a biophysical profile? _____

_____

_____

CRITICAL THINKING AND APPLICATION EXERCISES

1. Observe an amniocentesis. Prepare an oral presentation for your fellow classmates detailing nursing care before, during, and after the procedure.

2. Develop a patient-specific instruction sheet for a patient experiencing urinary frequency and urgency.

3. Create sample menus of a well-balanced diet for a pregnant patient based on the nutritional needs associated with pregnancy.

CHAPTER

Complications and High-Risk Conditions of the Prenatal Period

LEARNING OBJECTIVES

After studying this chapter, you should be able to:

♦ Describe potential complications of pregnancy.

♦ Identify the role of the nurse when caring for a patient whose pregnancy is complicated.

♦ Describe the impact of preexisting medical conditions upon pregnancy.

CHAPTER OVERVIEW

Many women experience complications or are placed at high risk during pregnancy as the result of either a preexisting condition or from the pregnancy itself. These problems may place both the mother and fetus at risk. Nursing care focuses on minimizing the risk to the mother and fetus and ensuring the best possible outcome.

◆ I. Introduction

A. Complications during pregnancy
  1. During pregnancy, some women experience problems due to known or unknown causes
  2. These conditions are a direct result of the pregnancy
  3. Other women have preexisting conditions that may affect the course of the pregnancy and the fetus
  4 Still other factors may contribute to placing the mother and fetus at risk

B. Factors placing patient at high risk
  1. Maternal age
    a. 16 years or younger
    b. Nullipara age 35 and older
    c. Multipara age 40 and older
  2. Parity (with at least one of the following):
    a. Eight years or more since last pregnancy
    b. High parity (five or more pregnancies of at least 20 weeks' duration)
    c. Pregnancy occurring within 3 months of last delivery
  3. Presence of chronic or acute medical conditions
  4. Poor past obstetric history
    a. Two or more premature deliveries
    b. Two or more consecutive miscarriages
    c. One or more stillbirths at term
    d. One or more gross anomalies
    e. Previous birth defects
    f. History of DYSTOCIA
    g. Poor self-care practices

◆ II. Hyperemesis gravidarum

A. Definition: pernicious vomiting during pregnancy

B. Pathophysiology: linked to trophoblastic activity, gonadotropin production, and psychological factors

C. Clinical manifestations
  1. Electrolyte imbalance
  2. Dehydration
  3. Oliguria
  4. Metabolic acidosis
  5. Jaundice

D. Management
  1. Restoration of fluid and electrolyte balance
  2. Control of vomiting
  3. Maintenance of adequate nutrition and rest

♦ III. Gestational trophoblastic disease

A. Definition

1. Developmental anomaly of the placenta that converts the chorionic villi into a mass of clear vesicles; also called molar pregnancy
2. There are two types: complete moles in which there is neither an embryo nor amniotic sac, and partial mole in which there is an embryo (usually with multiple abnormalities) and amniotic sac

B. Pathophysiology

1. Exact cause is unknown
2. Researchers believe condition may be associated with poor maternal nutrition or a defective ovum

C. Clinical manifestations

1. Disproportionate enlargement of the uterus
2. Excessive nausea and vomiting
3. Intermittent or continuous bright red or brownish vaginal bleeding by the 12th week of gestation
4. Symptoms of pregnancy-induced hypertension before the 20th week of gestation
5. No fetal heart tones
6. No fetal skeleton detected by ultrasound
7. Human chorionic gonadotropin (hCG) levels much higher than normal

D. Management

1. Induced abortion if a spontaneous one does not occur
2. Follow-up care vital because of increased risk of neoplasm
3. Weekly monitoring of hCG levels until they remain normal for three consecutive weeks
4. Periodic follow-up for one to two years
5. Pelvic examinations and chest X-rays at regular intervals
6. Emotional support for the couple, who are grieving for the lost pregnancy and an unsure obstetric and medical future
7. Advised to avoid pregnancy until hCG levels are normal (may take up to a year)

♦ IV. Placenta previa

A. Definition

1. Implantation of the placenta in the lower uterine segment (low implantation)
2. Possibly occluding the cervical os partially (partial placenta previa) or totally (total placenta previa)

B. Pathophysiology

1. Associated with uterine fibroid tumors and uterine scars from surgery

Placenta previa

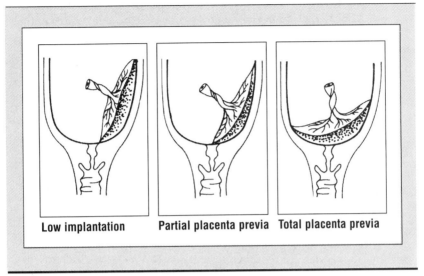

Low implantation   Partial placenta previa   Total placenta previa

    2. Placental villi are torn from the uterine wall as the lower uterine segment contracts and dilates in the third trimester

    3. Uterine sinuses are exposed at the placental site and bleeding occurs

C. Clinical manifestation

    1. Painless, bright red vaginal bleeding, especially during the third trimester

    2. Initially, scant bleeding but may increase with each successive incident

D. Management

    1. Depends upon when the first episode occurred and the amount of bleeding

    2. Limiting maternal activities

    3. Monitoring all relevant vital signs

CLINICAL ALERT

    4. Providing emotional support

    5. Note: rectal or vaginal exams, which could stimulate uterine activity, should not be performed unless equipment is available for vaginal and cesarean delivery; the placenta can be located via ultrasound

◆ V. Abruptio placentae

A. Definition

    1. Premature separation of the placenta from the uterine wall after 20 to 24 weeks of pregnancy

    2. May occur as late as during first or second stage of labor

B. Pathophysiology
   1. Primary cause is unknown
   2. Contributing factors include multiple pregnancy, hydramnios, cocaine use, decreased blood flow to the placenta, and trauma to the abdomen; women with low serum folic acid levels, vascular or renal disease, or pregnancy-induced hypertension are at risk

C. Clinical manifestations
   1. Hemorrhage, either concealed or apparent, with dark red vaginal bleeding
   2. Shock
   3. Acute abdominal pain
   4. Rigid abdomen
   5. Uteroplacental insufficiency

D. Management
   1. Monitor maternal vital signs, fetal heart rate, uterine contractions, and vaginal bleeding
   2. Evaluate maternal laboratory values
   3. Assess fluid and electrolyte balance
   4. Provide emotional support

E. Labor implications
   1. Likelihood of vaginal delivery depends on the degree and timing of separation in labor
   2. Cesarean delivery is indicated in moderate to severe placental separation
   3. Degree of placental separation can be graded from 0 to 3 to determine the fetal and maternal outcome (see *Grading abruptio placentae*)

F. Fetal implications
   1. Perinatal mortality depends on the degree of placental separation and fetal level of maturity
   2. Most serious complications stem from hypoxia, prematurity, and anemia

**CLINICAL
ALERT**

G. Maternal implications
   1. Mortality is approximately 6% and depends on the severity of the bleeding, the presence of coagulation defects, hypofibrinogenemia, and the time lapse between placental separation and delivery
   2. Postpartum patients are at risk for vascular spasm, intravascular clotting or hemorrhage, and renal failure from shock

Grading abruptio placentae

Separation of the placenta from the uterine wall is classified as minimal, moderate, or extreme. As the accompanying illustrations suggest, hemorrhaging may or may not be apparent, even with complete separation.

GRADE	CRITERIA
0	Maternal and fetal signs do not indicate difficulty. Premature separation is not apparent until the placenta is examined after delivery.
1	Minimal separation causes vaginal bleeding and alterations in maternal vital signs, but hemorrhagic shock and fetal distress do not appear.
2	Moderate separation produces signs of fetal distress. The uterus is tense and painful when palpated.
3	Extreme separation occurs, possibly causing maternal shock and fetal death without immediate intervention.

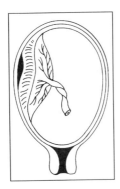 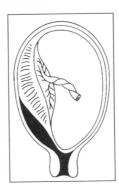 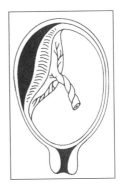

Partial separation
(Concealed hemorrhage)

Complete separation
(Apparent hemorrhage)

Complete separation
(Concealed hemorrhage)

◆ VI. Placenta accreta

A. Definition: attachment of chorionic villi onto or into the myometrium

B. Pathophysiology
1. Failure of the decidua (uterine lining during pregnancy) to develop in the placental bed
2. Allows for direct contact of placental tissue with the myometrium

C. Clinical manifestations
1. Maternal hemorrhage
2. Prolonged third stage of labor

D. Management: hysterectomy may be necessary, depending upon the amount of placental involvement

♦ VII. POLYHYDRAMNIOS (hydramnios)

A. Definition
1. Abnormally large amount (more than 2,000 ml) of amniotic fluid in the uterus
2. Fluid may have increased gradually (chronic type) or rapidly (acute type)

B. Pathophysiology
1. Exact cause unknown in about 35% of all cases
2. May be associated with diabetes mellitus (about 25%), erythroblastosis (about 10%), multiple gestation (about 10%), and congenital anomalies (about 20%)

C. Clinical manifestations
1. Depend upon the length of gestation, the amount of amniotic fluid, and whether the disorder is chronic or acute
2. Mild symptoms include abdominal discomfort and slight dyspnea
3. Severe symptoms include severe dyspnea, orthopnea, and edema of the vulva, legs, and abdomen
4. Symptoms common to mild and severe cases include uterine enlargement greater than expected for the length of gestation, and difficulty in outlining the fetal parts and in detecting fetal heart tones

D. Management
1. High-protein, low-sodium diet
2. Mild sedation
3. Amniocentesis to remove excess fluid
4. Induction of labor if the fetus is mature and symptoms are severe

E. Fetal-neonatal implications
1. Prolapsed umbilical cord at the rupture of membranes
2. Increased incidence of malpresentations
3. Increased perinatal mortality from fetal malformations and premature deliveries

F. Maternal implications
1. Shortness of breath, especially when the fluid exceeds 3,000 ml
2. Edema of legs from compression of the venae cavae
3. Increased incidence of postpartum hemorrhage

◆ **VIII. O**LIGOHYDRAMNIOS

    A. Definition: severely reduced and highly concentrated amniotic fluid

    B. Pathophysiology: associated with postmature infants, intrauterine growth retardation, and renal agenesis or obstruction in the fetal urinary tract

    C. Clinical manifestations: diagnosis made via ultrasonography

    D. Management: close medical supervision and fetal monitoring

    E. Fetal-neonatal implications
       1. Associated with renal anomalies
       2. Wrinkled, leathery skin
       3. Pulmonary hypoplasia
       4. Increased skeletal deformities
       5. Fetal hypoxia

    F. Maternal implications: prolonged, dysfunctional labor usually beginning before term

◆ **IX. Ectopic pregnancy**

    A. Definition
       1. Implantation of the fertilized ovum outside the uterine cavity
       2. Most ectopic pregnancies occur in a fallopian tube; other sites include the cervix, ovary, or abdominal cavity

    B. Pathophysiology
       1. Any condition that prevents or retards the passage of a fertilized ovum through the fallopian tube, such as hormonal factors, tubal damage from previous pelvic or tubal surgery, damage from pelvic inflammatory disease, tubal atony, tubal spasms, and malformed fallopian tubes
       2. Second most frequent cause of vaginal bleeding during pregnancy

    C. Clinical manifestations
       1. Irregular vaginal bleeding and dull abdominal pain on the affected side early in the pregnancy
       2. Abnormally low hCG titers
       3. Rupture of tubes, causing sudden and severe abdominal pain, syncope, and referred shoulder pain as the abdomen fills with blood; nausea and vomiting; shock with profuse hemorrhage

    D. Management
       1. Laparascopic removal of the ruptured tube (salpingectomy)
       2. Incision into the tube to remove the pregnancy (salpingostomy)
       3. Methotrexate to stop the trophoblastic cells from growing

4. Careful follow-up of hCG levels at regular intervals
5. Emotional support for parents grieving over the loss of the pregnancy

♦ X. Rh sensitization

A. Definition: antigen-antibody immunologic reaction within the body that occurs when an Rh-negative pregnant patient carries an Rh-positive fetus

B. Pathophysiology
1. Fetal red blood cells enter the maternal circulation and stimulate the production of Rh antibodies
2. In subsequent pregnancies, antibodies cross the placenta and enter the fetal circulation, causing erythroblastosis if the fetus is Rh positive

C. Clinical manifestations: increased concentration (optical density) of bilirubin and red blood cell breakdown products in the amniotic fluid

D. Management
1. Monitoring of the indirect Coombs' test (measures the amount of antibodies in the maternal blood)
2. Delta optical density analysis of the amniotic fluid at 26 weeks
3. Intrauterine transfusion
4. Emotional support to the parents

CLINICAL ALERT

5. Possible early delivery of the fetus
6. Administration of Rh$_o$(D) immunoglobulin at 28 weeks' gestation and within 72 hours following delivery of Rh positive infant to attain passive antibody protection for future pregnancies

♦ XI. Cystitis

A. Definition: inflammation of the lower urinary tract

B. Pathophysiology: caused by vesicoureteral reflux, urine stasis, and compression of the ureters

C. Clinical manifestations
1. Burning on urination
2. Urinary urgency and frequency
3. Temperature of 101° F (38.3° C)

D. Management
1. Proper perineal hygiene
2. Increased fluid intake
3. Urine culture to identify organism

4. Medication therapy
    a. Oral sulfonamides may be used in early pregnancy; use in later pregnancy can cause neonatal hyperbilirubinemia and kernicterus
    b. Ampicillin (Amcill) and nitrofurantoin (Furadantin) are appropriate in later pregnancy

◆ XII. Pyelonephritis

A. Definition: inflammation of the upper urinary tract

B. Pathophysiology
1. Ureteritis
2. Edema of the renal parenchyma
3. Ureteral swelling

C. Clinical manifestations
1. Severe colicky pain
2. Vomiting
3. Dehydration
4. Sudden onset with chills
5. Temperature of 103° to 105° F (39.4° to 40.6° C)
6. Flank pain

D. Management
1. Urine culture
2. Hospitalization
3. I.V. antibiotics
4. Monitoring of fluid intake and output
5. Vital signs
6. Laboratory reports
7. Monitoring fetal status

◆ XIII. Monilial infections

A. Definition: vaginal yeast infection

B. Causative organism: *Candida albicans*

C. Clinical manifestations
1. Thick, white, pruritic vaginal discharge
2. Dysuria and dyspareunia

D. Management
1. Drug therapy (nystatin [Mycostatin], clotrimazole [Lotrimin]),
2. Review of personal hygiene
3. Condom use or abstinence from intercourse until infection is cured

CLINICAL ALERT

E. Fetal-neonatal implications: if infection is not cured before delivery, the fetus may contract thrush by direct contact with the organism in the vagina

F. Patient at risk: one with poorly controlled diabetes mellitus or on steroid or antibiotic therapy

◆ XIV. Miscarriage (spontaneous abortion)

A. Definition
   1. Spontaneous termination of a pregnancy before the 20th week of gestation
   2. May be threatened, imminent, and incomplete, or complete

B. Pathophysiology
   1. More than 50% are caused by abnormalities in fetoplacental development
   2. Remainder are from maternal or unknown causes

C. Clinical manifestations
   1. Symptom severity depends on the gestational age at the time of miscarriage
   2. Symptoms include uterine cramping; vaginal bleeding; weakly positive urine pregnancy test; minimal or absent estrogen, hCG, and progesterone titers

D. Management: varies with type and stage of spontaneous abortion (see *Managing spontaneous abortion*)

◆ XV. Pregnancy-induced hypertension (PIH)

A. Definition
   1. Pregnancy disorder characterized by hypertension, proteinuria, and edema
   2. Can be categorized as preeclampsia (before seizures) and eclampsia (with seizures)

B. Pathophysiology: predisposing factors include diabetes mellitus, malnutrition, adolescent mother, hydramnios, hypertension, renal disease, obesity, multiple pregnancy, hydatidiform mole, and familial tendency

C. Clinical manifestations
   a. Hypertension: defined as blood pressure over 140/90 mm Hg
   b. Proteinuria: measured as 0.5 g/liter/day, or +1 or +2 via dipstick
   c. Increase in generalized edema associated with a sudden weight gain of greater than 5 lb (2.3 kg) per week
   d. Usually appears between the 20th and 24th weeks of gestation and disappears within 42 days after delivery
   e. A final diagnosis usually deferred until blood pressure returns to normal after delivery; if blood pressure remains elevated, chronic hypertension, either alone or superimposed on (PIH), may be the cause

Managing spontaneous abortion

TYPE OR STAGE	MANAGEMENT
Threatened miscarriage	Limit the patient's activities for 24 to 48 hours. Restrict coitus for approximately 2 weeks.
Imminent and incomplete abortion	Assist with dilatation and curettage to ensure emptying of the uterus.
Complete abortion	If the uterus emptied on its own and the patient has no signs of infection, no further intervention is needed

    f. Additional manifestations: increased blood urea nitrogen, creatinine, and uric acid levels; frontal headaches; blurred vision; hyperreflexia; nausea; vomiting; irritability; cerebral disturbances; and epigastric pain

D. Maternal implications

    1. Disorder may progress to seizures (eclampsia)

    2. Maternal mortality rate in eclampsia is 10% to 15%, usually resulting from intracranial hemorrhage and congestive heart failure

E. Severe complications of eclampsia: cerebral edema, maternal cerebrovascular accident, abruptio placentae with or without disseminated intravascular coagulation, and fetal death

F. Management

    1. High-protein diet, with restriction of excessively salty foods

    2. Bed rest in a lateral position

    3. Close observance of blood pressure, fetal heart rate, edema, proteinuria, and signs of pending eclampsia

CLINICAL ALERT

    4. Administration of magnesium sulfate, a neuromuscular sedative that reduces the amount of acetylcholine produced by motor nerves, thus preventing seizures (urine output must be at least 30 ml/hour because 99% of the drug is excreted by the kidneys)

       a. Signs of magnesium sulfate toxicity must be promptly identified and management initiated.

       b. These signs and symptoms include elevated serum levels, decreased deep tendon reflexes, muscle flaccidity, central nervous system depression, and decreased respiratory rate and renal function

       c. The antidote to magnesium sulfate is calcium gluconate

♦ XVI. Incompetent cervix

A. Definition
  1. Painless premature dilation of the cervix
  2. Generally occurs in the 4th to 5th month of gestation

B. Pathophysiology
  1. Associated with congenital structural defects or previous cervical trauma resulting from surgery or delivery
  2. Also associated with increased maternal age

C. Clinical manifestations
  1. History of repeated second trimester miscarriages
  2. Cervical dilation in the absence of contractions/pain
  3. Possible rupture of membranes and discharge of amniotic fluid

D. Management
  1. Placement of a purse-string suture, known as a cerclage, in the cervix to help keep the cervix closed until term or the patient goes into labor.
  2. Removal of suture at about 37 to 39 weeks
  3. Emotional support

♦ XVII. Diabetes

A. Definition: a disorder of fat, carbohydrate, and protein metabolism caused by a relative or complete lack of insulin secretion by pancreatic beta cells
  1. Insulin-dependent diabetes mellitus (IDDM) predates the pregnancy
  2. Gestational diabetes mellitus, a form of non-insulin-dependent diabetes mellitus, may begin at pregnancy

B. Pathophysiology
  1. Gestational diabetes mellitus occurs when the patient's pancreas, stressed by the normal adaptations to pregnancy, cannot meet the increased demands for insulin
  2. The age of onset and the duration of pre-existing diabetes mellitus, not the daily insulin requirements, are crucial factors related to outcome

C. Clinical manifestations
  1. All non-IDDM pregnant women screened at 26 to 28 weeks with a 50-g, 1-hour glucose test.
  2. If the results are abnormal (130 mg), a 3-hour glucose tolerance test performed
  3. If two or more values are abnormal, the patient is diagnosed with gestational diabetes

TEACHING TIPS
Pregnant patient with diabetes

Be sure to include the following topics in your teaching plan for the pregnant patient with diabetes:
- Explanation of diabetes
- Procedure for fingerstick blood sugar monitoring
- Frequency of blood sugar monitoring
- Insulin requirements
- Insulin administration technique
- Insulin action, dosage, frequency, and possible effects
- Possible danger signs
- Implications for mother and fetus
- Dietary restrictions
- Activity and exercise precautions
- Regular checkups and diagnostic testing
- Need for compliance and follow-up

D. Management
   1. Gestational diabetes mellitus
      a. Blood glucose levels should be monitored four times/day; fasting blood sugar (FBS) and 2 hours postprandial
      b. Target glucose levels for FBS <100 mg and postprandial <120 mg.
      c. Careful monitoring of diet, exercise, and insulin administration and patient education

CLINICAL ALERT

      d. Oral hypoglycemic agents are contraindicated in pregnancy because of their adverse effects on the fetus and newborn

CLINICAL ALERT

   2. Insulin-dependent diabetes
      a. Close monitoring of glucose levels because of tendency for wide fluctuations in blood glucose levels
      b. In general, insulin requirements decrease during the first trimester and increase during second and third trimesters

E. Maternal implications: the patient with gestational diabetes has a 30% to 40% chance of developing diabetes mellitus in 1 to 25 years

F. Fetal-neonatal implications
   1. Insulin-dependent diabetes is associated with an increased risk of congenital anomalies, hydramnios, macrosomia, PIH, spontaneous abortion, and fetal death
   2. A condition unique to the infant of an insulin-dependent diabetic is sacral agenesis, a congenital anomaly characterized by incomplete formation of the spinal column

◆ XVIII. Sickle-cell anemia

A. Definition: a recessive autosomal disorder in which red blood cells become sickle-shaped

B. Pathophysiology: vascular obstruction in the capillaries leads to anemia

C. Maternal implications: increased incidence of PIH, urinary tract infections, congestive heart failure, pneumonia, pulmonary infarction, crisis, and postpartum hemorrhage

D. Fetal-neonatal implications: risk for intrauterine growth retardation and perinatal fetal death from spontaneous abortion and prematurity in a patient with sickle-cell anemia

E. Management
1. Monitor hemoglobin and hematocrit values
2. Avoid contributing factors, such as dehydration, stress, hypoxia, infection, acidosis, and sudden cooling
3. Monitor for thrombophlebitis (positive HOMANS' SIGN)
4. Provide folic acid supplements to decrease erythropoietic demands and capillary stasis
5. Administer heparin, if prescribed; warfarin (Coumadin) is contraindicated because it can cross the placenta and harm the fetus

CLINICAL
ALERT

◆ XIX. Heart disease

A. Definition
1. Impaired cardiac function
2. Primarily from congenital or rheumatic heart disease
   a. Congenital heart disease: atrial septal defect, ventricular septal defect, pulmonary stenosis, coarctation of the aorta
   b. Rheumatic heart disease: endocarditis with scar tissue formation on the mitral, aortic, or tricuspid valves with resulting stenosis or regurgitation

B. Pathophysiology: problem depends on the defect's location and severity
1. Valvular stenosis decreases blood flow through the valve, increasing the workload on heart chambers located before the stenotic valve
2. Regurgitation permits blood to leak through an incompletely closed valve, increasing the workload on heart chambers on either side of the affected valve

C. Clinical manifestations
1. Dyspnea
2. Tachycardia
3. Diastolic murmur at the heart's apex

Heart disease and pregnancy

A patient with heart disease may or may not experience a difficult pregnancy; success depends on the type and extent of the disease, as shown below. A patient in Class I or II usually completes a successful pregnancy and delivery without major complications. One in Class III must maintain complete bed rest to complete the pregnancy. One in Class IV is a poor candidate for pregnancy.

CLASS	DESCRIPTION
I	The patient has unrestricted physical activity. Ordinary activity causes no discomfort, cardiac insufficiency, or anginal pain.
II	The patient has a slight limitation on physical activity. Ordinary activity causes excessive fatigue, palpitations, dyspnea, or anginal pain.
III	The patient has a moderate to marked limitation on activity. With less than ordinary activity, she experiences excessive fatigue, palpitations, dyspnea, or anginal pain.
IV	The patient cannot engage in any physical activity without discomfort. Cardiac insufficiency or anginal pain occurs even at rest.

    4. Cough

    5. Hemoptysis

    6. Crackles at the lungs' bases

D. Maternal implications: stress on the cardiopulmonary system (see also Chapter 4, II, A)

    1. The normal heart can compensate for increased demands, but if myocardial or valvular disease develops, or if the patient has a congenital heart defect, cardiac decompensation may occur

    2. A patient with a cardiac disorder is at greatest risk when blood volume peaks between the 28th and 32nd week of gestation

    3. Note: successfully delivering a healthy baby depends on the type and extent of the disease (see *Heart disease and pregnancy*)

E. Fetal-neonatal implications: decreased placental perfusion leading to intrauterine growth retardation, fetal distress, or prematurity

F. Management: limiting activities, close medical supervision, adequate rest, limited sodium intake, and antibiotics as prophylactic measures

CLINICAL ALERT

◆ XX. Substance abuse

A. Definition
   1. The misuse, or overuse of substances, including alcohol, prescription, over-the-counter, and illicit drugs
   2. During pregnancy, most commonly associated with alcohol and illicit drugs
   3. The number of substance abusers has increased during the last decade

B. Pathophysiology
   1. Depends on substance abused
   2. Causes fetal harm; most detrimental when used during first trimester when fetal organs being formed

C. Clinical manifestations
   1. The majority of pregnant addicts do not seek prenatal care
   2. Substance abuse may be compounded by malnutrition, alcoholism, sexually transmitted diseases, or poor self-image
   3. Maternal complications include cellulitis, septic phlebitis, superficial abscesses, and acute pulmonary edema

D. Fetal-neonatal implications (see also Chapter 9, VII and VIII)
   1. Management depends on substance being abused
   2. An addicted patient should receive long-term counseling and rehabilitation (social, medical, psychiatric, and vocational)
   3. The majority of substance abusers are polysubstance abusers, making it difficult to predict maternal-fetal-neonatal implications resulting from synergistic effects

POINTS TO REMEMBER

◆ Placenta previa is marked by painless, bright red vaginal bleeding, while a woman with abruptio placenta generally experiences acute abdominal pain with either an apparent or concealed hemorrhage.

◆ Pregnancy-induced hypertension is characterized by hypertension, proteinuria, and edema.

◆ The woman with hydramnios is at increased risk for prolapsed cord at the time of rupture of membranes.

◆ The fetus of a substance-abusing mother is at most risk of harm during the first trimester.

STUDY QUESTIONS

To evaluate your understanding of this chapter, answer the following questions in the space provided; then compare your responses with the correct answers in Appendix B, page 173.

1. Which factors place a woman at increased risk for a complicated pregnancy?

   _____

   _____

2. What are three factors that characterize pregnancy-induced hypertension?

   _____

   _____

3. Which procedure is used to manage a patient with an incompetent cervix?

   _____

   _____

CRITICAL THINKING AND APPLICATION EXERCISES

1. Interview an adolescent pregnant patient. Develop a patient-specific plan of care addressing this patient's high-risk needs.

2. Follow a patient considered high risk or experiencing a complication throughout the prenatal period. Develop a patient-specific plan of care including any needs for monitoring, follow-up, and education.

Normal Labor and Delivery

LEARNING OBJECTIVES

After studying this chapter, you should be able to:

♦ Differentiate among the four stages of labor.

♦ State the nurse's role when caring for a patient in labor.

♦ Describe a pregnant patient's physiologic and psychological responses to labor.

♦ Identify methods of assessing fetal status during labor.

♦ Describe current theories of pain.

♦ Identify potential sources of pain during labor and delivery.

♦ Name the pharmacologic and nonpharmacologic methods used to relieve pain during labor and delivery.

♦ Discuss the nurse's role in caring for a patient who has received analgesics or anesthesia during labor and delivery.

♦ Describe potential maternal, fetal, and neonatal adverse reactions to pharmacologic measures used during labor and delivery.

CHAPTER OVERVIEW

Throughout labor, many physiologic events occur, resulting in the delivery of the neonate. Specific signs indicate the onset of labor; as the patient progresses, various physiologic and psychosocial responses occur. Throughout labor and delivery, the patient and fetus are monitored closely to ensure the optimal outcome for both. If necessary, obstetric procedures, analgesia, and anesthetics may be used.

♦ I. Theories about labor initiation

A. Oxytocin stimulation
   1. Researchers have not proven that either maternal or fetal oxytocin initiates labor
   2. It is believed that the myometrium of a patient at term is increasingly sensitive to oxytocin, possibly because of estrogen's stimulating effects

B. Progesterone withdrawal
   1. Decreased progesterone metabolism in the fetus (and possibly in the pregnant patient) may stimulate prostaglandin synthesis in the chorioamnion
   2. This results in increased uterine contractility

C. Estrogen stimulation
   1. Estrogen irritates the myometrium and promotes prostaglandin synthesis
   2. This increases myometrial muscle contraction and helps transmit impulses over the uterine muscle after the muscle cells are irritated and the muscle contracts

D. Fetal cortisol: cortisol may alter the biochemistry of the fetal membrane

E. Distention
   1. The uterus stretches
   2. As a result, the production, release, and myometrial concentrations of prostaglandin F increase

F. Fetal membrane phospholipid–arachidonic acid–prostaglandin
   1. Prostaglandin is a biocompound present in blood and amniotic fluid
   2. It stimulates the smooth muscle of the myometrium to contract

◆ II. Components of labor

A. General information
   1. Three important components of labor—the passage, passenger, and power (3 P's)—must work together for labor to progress normally
   2. If any one of these components is altered, the outcome of labor can be adversely affected
   3. Other factors associated with the patient and placenta also may affect labor

B. The Passage
   1. Refers to maternal pelvis and soft tissues
   2. Affected by the following factors
      a. Shape of the inlet
         (1) Gynecoid: round (about 50% of female pelvices)
         (2) Anthropoid: oval (about 25% of female pelvices)
         (3) Android: heart-shaped, like the normal male pelvis (about 20% of female pelvices)
         (4) Platypelloid: transverse oval (about 5% of female pelvices)
      b. Structure of pelvis
         (1) Pelvic joints
            (a) Symphysis pubis
            (b) Right sacroiliac joint
            (c) Left sacroiliac joint
            (d) Sacrococcygeal joint
         (2) Pelvic bones
            (a) Ilium
            (b) Ischium
            (c) Sacrum
            (d) Coccyx
         (3) True versus false pelvis
            (a) The false pelvis is that portion above the pelvic inlet
            (b) The true pelvis consists of the pelvic inlet, pelvic cavity, and pelvic outlet
      c. Pelvic diameters
         (1) Inlet: anteroposterior diameters
            (a) True conjugate: 4⅜″ (11 cm) or greater
            (b) Diagonal conjugate: 4⅞″ to 5⅛″ (12.5 to 13 cm)
            (c) Obstetric conjugate: 4⅞″ to 5⅛″
         (2) Inlet: transverse diameter: 5⅜″ (13.5 cm) or greater
         (3) Inlet: oblique diameter: 5″ (12.7 cm) or greater

Head diameters at term

The illustration below depicts three commonly used measurements of fetal head diameters. The measurements are averages for term neonates. Individual measurements vary with fetal size, attitude, and presentation.

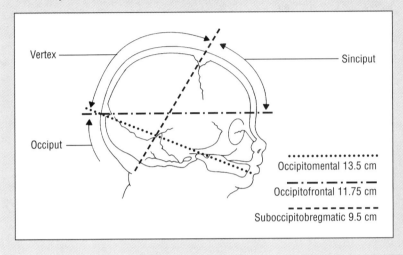

Vertex

Sinciput

Occiput

Occipitomental 13.5 cm

Occipitofrontal 11.75 cm

Suboccipitobregmatic 9.5 cm

(4) Outlet
    (a) Anteroposterior diameter: approximately 4⅝″ (11.7 cm)
    (b) Transverse or intertuberous diameter: 3⅞″ to 5⅜″ (10 to 13.7 cm)
    (c) Posterior sagittal diameter: approximately 3½″ (9 cm)
  d. Soft tissues
    (1) Lower uterine segment: segment of the uterus that expands to accommodate intrauterine contents as the walls of the upper segment thicken
    (2) Cervix: the cervix is drawn up and over the presenting part as it descends
    (3) Vaginal canal: the vagina distends to accommodate the fetus
C. Passenger
  1. Refers to ability of fetus to move through the passage
  2. Affected by fetal features
    a. Fetal skull
      (1) Size
        (a) The smallest diameter enters the pelvis first
        (b) The head can flex or extend 45 degrees and rotate 180 degrees, which allows its smallest diameters to move down

Molding of the head: Cephalic presentations

In a cephalic presentation, the skull molds to adapt to an unyielding maternal pelvis. The degree of head flexion or extension dictates which head diameter enters the pelvis first. The illustrations below show possible cephalic presentations; dotted lines indicate molding.

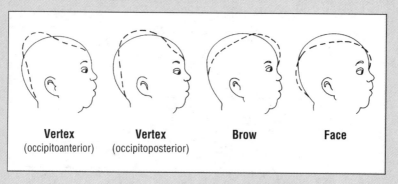

| **Vertex** | **Vertex** | **Brow** | **Face** |
| (occipitoanterior) | (occipitoposterior) | | |

the birth canal and pass through the maternal pelvis (see *Head diameters at term*)
 (2) Shape
  (a) Pressure is exerted by the maternal pelvis and birth canal during labor and delivery
  (b) In response, the sutures of the skull allow the cranial bones to shift, resulting in MOLDING of the fetal head (see *Molding of the head: Cephalic presentations*)
 b. Lie: relationship of the long axis (spine) of the fetus to the long axis of the mother
  (1) Longitudinal lie: the long axis of the fetus is parallel to the long axis of the mother
  (2) Transverse lie: the long axis of the fetus is perpendicular to the long axis of the mother
 c. Presentation: portion of the fetus that enters the pelvic passageway first
  (1) Cephalic: vertex, brow, and face
  (2) Breech: frank, single or double footling, and complete
  (3) Shoulder: transverse lie that must be turned before delivery
 d. Attitude: relationship of the fetal parts to one another

Fetal positions

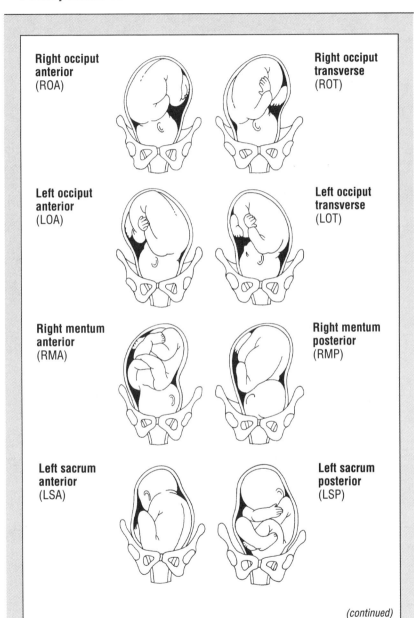

Right occiput anterior (ROA)

Right occiput transverse (ROT)

Left occiput anterior (LOA)

Left occiput transverse (LOT)

Right mentum anterior (RMA)

Right mentum posterior (RMP)

Left sacrum anterior (LSA)

Left sacrum posterior (LSP)

(continued)

Fetal positions (continued)

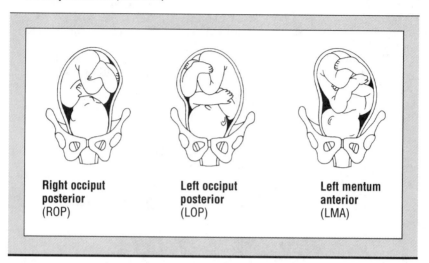

| Right occiput posterior (ROP) | Left occiput posterior (LOP) | Left mentum anterior (LMA) |

    e. Position: relationship of the landmark on the presenting part to the front, back, and sides of the maternal pelvis (see *Fetal positions*); notations used to designate fetal position include the following:

        (1) Side of maternal pelvis: right (R) or left (L)

        (2) Landmark on the presenting part: occiput (O), mentum (M), sacrum (S), acromion process (A)

        (3) Position of the landmark on the pelvis: anterior (A), posterior (P), transverse (T)

        (4) Positions in vertex presentations: ROA, ROT, ROP, LOA, LOT, LOP

        (5) Positions in face presentation: RMA, RMT, RMP, LMA, LMT, LMP

        (6) Positions in breech presentation: RSA, RST, RSP, LSA, LST, LSP

D. Power

    1. Refers to uterine contractions

    2. Causes complete cervical effacement and dilation (see Section IX in this chapter for more information)

E. Other factors

    1. Mother's ability to bear down (voluntary use of abdominal muscles to push during the second stage of labor)

    2. Placental positioning (see Chapter 4, XIII, C)

    3. Psychological readiness

        a. Support systems

        b. Preparation for childbirth

Distinguishing between true and false labor

Knowing how to recognize the primary characteristics of true and false labor can help the nurse distinguish between the two conditions.

TRUE LABOR	FALSE LABOR
Regular contractions	Irregular contractions
Back discomfort that spreads to the abdomen	Discomfort that is localized in the abdomen
Progressive cervical dilation and effacement	No cervical change
Gradually shortened intervals between contractions	No change or irregular change
Increased intensity of contractions with ambulation	Contractions may be relieved with ambulation
Contractions that increase in duration and intensity	Usually no change in contractions

    c. Past experiences
    d. Coping mechanisms
    e. Accomplishment of the tasks of pregnancy

♦ III. Preliminary signs of labor

A. Lightening
    1. Fetal descent into the pelvis
    2. Usually occurring two to three weeks before term in a primiparous patient and later or during labor in a multiparous patient

B. Braxton Hicks contractions
    1. Occur irregularly and intermittently throughout pregnancy
    2. May become uncomfortable and produce false labor (see *Distinguishing between true and false labor*)

C. Cervical changes
    1. Usually occur several days before initiation of labor
    2. Cervix softens, begins to efface, and dilates slightly

D. Bloody show
    1. Mucus plug is expelled from the cervix
    2. Pink-tinged secretions result

E. Rupture of membranes (ROM)
  1. ROM occurs before onset of labor in approximately 12% of patients
  2. Labor begins within 24 hours for about 80% of these patients

F. Burst of energy
  1. Patient may experience a sudden burst of energy before the onset of labor
  2. This is commonly manifested by housecleaning activities and called the "nesting instinct"

♦ **IV. Stages of labor**

A. First stage
  1. The first stage is measured from the onset of true labor to complete DILATION of the cervix
  2. Duration usually ranges from 6 to 18 hours in a primiparous patient and from 2 to 10 hours in a multiparous patient
  3. It is divided into three phases: latent, active, and transitional
    a. Latent phase
       (1) Dilation measures 0 to 3 cm
       (2) Contractions are irregular
    b. Active phase
       (1) Dilation measures 4 to 7 cm
       (2) Contractions are approximately 5 to 8 minutes apart, last 45 to 60 seconds, and are moderate to strong in intensity
    c. Transitional phase
       (1) Dilation measures 8 to 10 cm
       (2) Contractions are approximately 1 to 2 minutes apart, last 60 to 90 seconds, and are strong in intensity

B. Second stage
  1. The second stage extends from complete dilation to delivery of fetus
  2. Duration usually ranges from 2 to 60 minutes, averaging about 40 minutes (20 contractions) for the primiparous patient and 20 minutes (10 contractions) for the multiparous patient
  3. Fetus is moved along the birth canal by mechanisms of labor
    a. Engagement: the fetus's head is considered engaged when the biparietal diameter passes the pelvic inlet
    b. Descent: movement of the presenting part through the pelvis
    c. Flexion: the head flexes so that the chin moves closer to the chest
    d. Internal rotation: rotation of the head to pass through the ischial spines
    e. Extension: extension of the head as it passes under the symphysis pubis
    f. External rotation: the head is externally rotated as the shoulders rotate to the anteroposterior position in the pelvis

C. Third stage
   1. The third stage extends from delivery of the neonate to expulsion of the placenta
   2. Duration ranges from 5 to 30 minutes

D. Fourth stage
   1. The fourth stage is the first hour after delivery
   2. Primary activity is promotion of maternal neonatal bonding

◆ V. Maternal physiologic responses to labor

A. Physiologic responses
   1. Cardiovascular system
      a. Increased intrathoracic pressure during pushing in the second stage
      b. Increased peripheral resistance during contractions, which elevates blood pressure and decreases pulse rate
      c. Increased cardiac output
   2. Fluid and electrolyte balance
      a. Increased water loss from diaphoresis and hyperventilation
      b. Increased evaporative water volume from increased respiratory rate
   3. Respiratory system
      a. Increased oxygen consumption
      b. Increased respiratory rate
   4. Hematopoietic system
      a. Increased plasma fibrinogen and leukocytes
      b. Decreased blood coagulation time and blood glucose levels
   5. Gastrointestinal system
      a. Decreased gastric motility and absorption
      b. Prolonged gastric emptying time
   6. Renal system
      a. Forward and upward displacement of the bladder base at engagement
      b. Possible proteinuria from muscle breakdown
      c. Possible impairment of blood and lymph drainage from the bladder base, resulting from edema caused by the presenting part

B. Psychological responses
   1. First stage
      a. The patient may feel anticipation, excitement, or apprehension
      b. During active phase, the patient becomes serious and concerned about the progress of labor; she may ask for pain medication or use breathing techniques
      c. During the transitional phase, the patient may lose control, thrash in bed, groan, or cry out

    2. Second stage

        a. Maternal behavior changes from coping with contractions to actively pushing

        b. Patient may become exhausted

    3. Third stage

        a. The patient typically focuses on the neonate's condition

        b. Patient may feel discomfort from uterine contractions before expelling the placenta

    4. Fourth stage

        a. The patient focuses on the neonate

        b. The primary activity is promotion of maternal-neonatal bonding

◆ VI. Nursing care during labor and delivery

A. Care during all four stages

    1. Provide emotional support to the patient and coach

    2. Monitor and record I.V. fluid intake, urine output, and vital signs

    3. Assess the need for pain medication, and evaluate the effectiveness of medication administered

    4. Maintain aseptic technique

    5. Maintain the patient's comfort by offering mouth care, ice chips, and a change of bed linen

    6. Explain the purpose of all nursing actions and medical equipment

B. During first and second stages

    1. Inform the patient of labor progress: dilation, STATION, EFFACEMENT, and fetal well-being (see Section VII in this chapter for more information)

    2. Monitor the frequency, duration, and intensity of contractions

    3. Monitor fetal heart rate during and between contractions, noting rate, accelerations, decelerations, and variability

CLINICAL ALERT

    4. Observe for rupture of membranes, noting the time, color, odor, amount, and consistency of amniotic fluid

    5. Observe for prolapsed cord and check the fetal heart rate immediately after rupture of membranes

    6. Assess for signs of hypotensive supine syndrome; if blood pressure falls:

        a. Position the patient on the left side

        b. Increase the primary I.V. flow rate

        c. Administer oxygen through a face mask at 6 to 10 liters/minute

C. During first, second, and third stages

    1. Assist with breathing techniques

    2. Encourage rest between contractions

Leopold's maneuvers

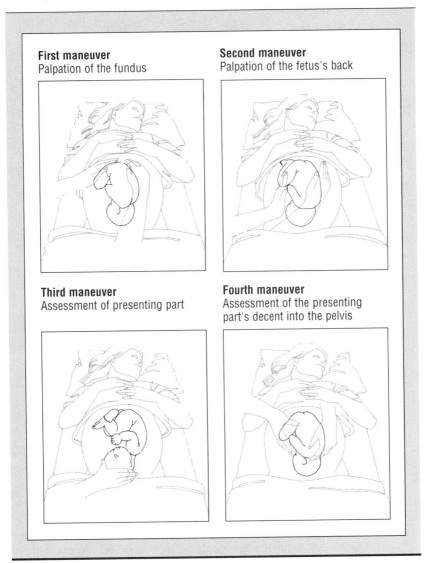

First maneuver
Palpation of the fundus

Second maneuver
Palpation of the fetus's back

Third maneuver
Assessment of presenting part

Fourth maneuver
Assessment of the presenting part's decent into the pelvis

    D. During second stage: observe the perineum for show and bulging

    E. During fourth stage
        1. Assess lochia, location and consistency of fundus, encourage bonding
        2. Initiate breast-feeding

◆ VII. Maternal evaluation during labor

A. Monitor the progress of labor

1. Dilation: opening of the external os from 0 to 10 cm
2. Effacement: cervical thinning and shortening, measured from 0% (thick) to 100% (paper thin)
3. Position and presenting part: using abdominal palpation (Leopold's maneuvers) determine fetal position and presentation (see *Leopold's maneuvers,* page 71)

   a. First maneuver: palpation of the fundus to identify the occupying fetal part; the fetus's head is firm and rounded and moves freely, whereas the breech is softer and less regular and moves with the trunk

   b. Second maneuver: abdominal palpation to identify the location of the fetus's back; the back feels firm, smooth, and convex, whereas the front is soft, irregular, and concave

   c. Third maneuver: grasping of the lower portion of the abdomen above the symphysis pubis to identify the fetal part presenting over the inlet; an unengaged head can be rocked from side to side; this maneuver helps determine the attitude of the head

   d. Fourth maneuver: movement of fingers down both sides of the uterus to assess the descent of the presenting part into the pelvis; as the fingers move downward, greater resistance will be met on the cephalic prominence (brow) side; this maneuver helps determine whether the head is flexed

4. Station: relationship of the presenting part to the pelvic ischial spines (see *Measuring fetal station*)

   a. Presenting part even with the ischial spines is at 0 station

   b. Presenting part above the ischial spines is -3, -2, or -1

   c. Presenting part below the ischial spines is +1, +2, or +3

B. Patient monitoring

1. Encourage the patient to void every 2 hours; a full bladder can impede fetal descent and cause dysfunctional labor
2. Monitor the patient for signs of dehydration, such as poor skin turgor, decreased urine output, and dry mucous membranes
3. Use an external pressure transducer to monitor the patient for tetanic contractions (sustained, prolonged contractions with little rest between)

Measuring fetal station

Fetal station, determined by vaginal examination, is the relationship of the presenting part to the ischial spines.

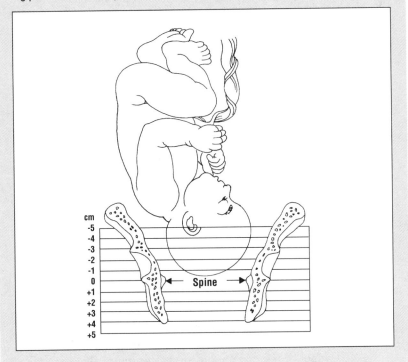

cm
-5
-4
-3
-2
-1
0 ←— Spine —→
+1
+2
+3
+4
+5

♦ VIII. Fetal evaluation during labor

A. External electronic monitoring

1. Types

   a. Noninvasive monitoring of fetal heart rate (FHR) either intermittently with a hand-held device or continuously with a large fetal monitor

   b. Continuous monitoring of contraction intensity and frequency with a tocodynamometer, a pressure device that, in response to uterine contractions, transfers an electrical impulse to the monitor and creates a readout

2. Advantages

   a. Evaluates decreased variability and periodic changes

   b. Grossly evaluates contractions

   c. Provides a permanent record

3. Disadvantages
   a. Is subject to artifacts (distortions in the readout)
   b. May be uncomfortable for the pregnant patient
   c. Cannot assess variability unless decreased
   d. May divert the nurse's attention from the patient

B. Internal electronic monitoring
   1. Types
      a. Internal spiral electrode
         (1) Is applied to the epidermis of the presenting part
         (2) Provides a continuous recording of the FHR
         (3) Demonstrates accurate baseline, true baseline variability, and periodic changes
      b. Intrauterine pressure catheter
         (1) Is inserted into the uterine cavity alongside the fetus
         (2) Continuously and accurately records the intensity and frequency of contractions
   2. Advantages
      a. Provides the most precise assessment of the FHR and uterine contractions
      b. Is not affected by changes in maternal or fetal positioning
   3. Disadvantages
      a. Increases the risk of maternal infection
      b. May cause a laceration or abscess if inserted into the fetal presenting part
      c. May limit maternal movement

CLINICAL ALERT

      d. May divert the nurse's attention from the pregnant patient
      e. Cannot be inserted until membranes rupture, the cervix dilates at least 1 cm, and the fetus descends

◆ IX. Uterine contractions

A. Phases
   1. Increment: the building-up phase and longest phase
   2. Acme: the peak of the contraction
   3. Decrement: the letting-down phase

B. Duration
   1. Is measured from the beginning of the increment to the end of the decrement
   2. Averages 30 seconds in early labor and 60 seconds in later labor

C. Frequency
   1. Is measured from the beginning of one contraction to the beginning of the next
   2. Averages 5 to 30 minutes apart in early labor and 2 to 3 minutes apart in later labor

Uterine contractions

As shown in the diagram below, uterine contractions occur in three phases: increment (building up), acme (peak), and decrement (letting down). Between contractions is a period of relaxation. The two most important features of contractions are duration and frequency. Duration is the elapsed time from the start to the end of one contraction. Frequency refers to the elapsed time from the start of one contraction to the start of the next contraction.

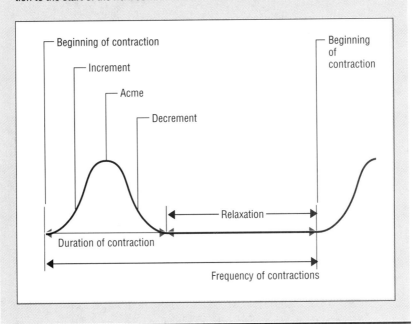

D. Intensity
   1. Is measured during the acme phase
   2. Can be measured with an intrauterine catheter or by palpation (normal resting pressure when using an intrauterine catheter is 5 to 15 mm Hg; pressure increases to 30 to 50 mm Hg during the acme)

◆ X. Fetal heart rate patterns

A. Decelerations of FHR
   1. Early
      a. Cause: head compression
      b. Shape: uniform, smooth waveforms that inversely mirror the corresponding contractions

Fetal heart rate decelerations

The monitor strips below show early, late, and variable decelerations of fetal heart rate, along with corresponding uterine contractions.

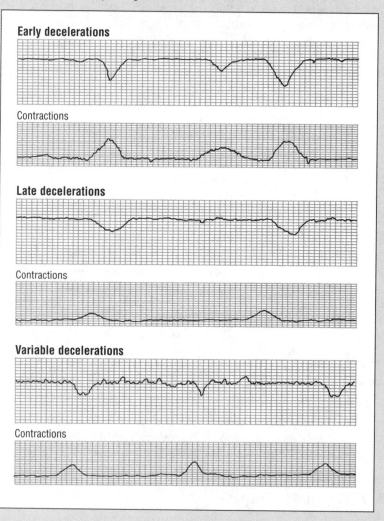

Early decelerations

Contractions

Late decelerations

Contractions

Variable decelerations

Contractions

c. Range: normal range of 120 to 160 beats/minute
d. Clinical significance: reassuring pattern; not associated with any fetal difficulties
e. Nursing interventions: none required

DECISION TREE
Evaluating fetal heart rate deceleration

Use the decision tree below when determining how to proceed should you identify fetal heart rate deceleration.

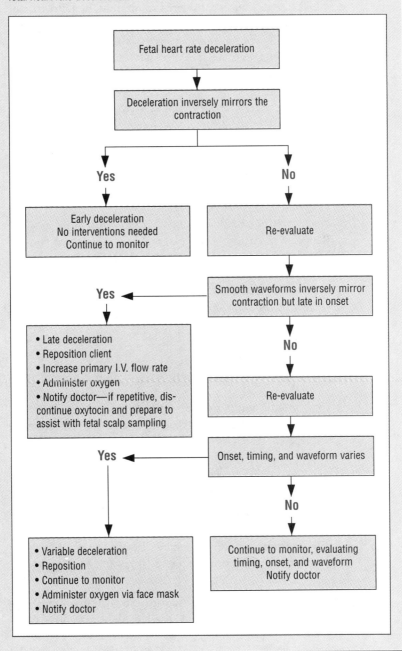

2. Late
   a. Cause: uteroplacental insufficiency
   b. Shape: smooth, uniform waveforms that inversely mirror the contractions but are late in their onset
   c. Range: usually within the normal range with a high baseline; may drop to below 100 beats/minute when severe
   d. Clinical significance: considered an ominous sign if persistent and uncorrected; pattern is associated with decreased Apgar scores, fetal hypoxia, and acidosis
   e. Nursing interventions
      (1) Place the patient in the left lateral position
      (2) Increase the primary I.V. flow rate
      (3) Administer oxygen through a face mask according to hospital protocol or the doctor's order (commonly 6 to 8 liters/minute)
      (4) Discontinue oxytocin infusion
      (5) Assist with fetal blood sampling, if ordered
3. Variable
   a. Cause: umbilical cord compression
   b. Shape: vary in onset, occurrence, and waveform
   c. Range: in severe cases, the heart rate may decelerate below 70 beats/minute for more than 30 seconds, with a slow return to baseline
   d. Clinical significance: occur in approximately 50% of labors and are usually transient and correctable; occurrences are not associated with low Apgar scores
   e. Nursing interventions
      (1) Administer oxygen through a face mask according to hospital protocol or the doctor's order (commonly 8 to 10 liters/minute)
      (2) Continue to monitor the FHR
      (3) Start amnioinfusion for repetitive variable decelerations, if ordered

B. Accelerations of FHR
   1. Cause: normally from fetal movements but also can occur with contractions
   2. Shape: uniform or variable
   3. Range: usually above 150 beats/minute
   4. Clinical significance: indicates fetal well-being
   5. Nursing interventions: none required

C. Variability of FHR
   1. Cause: normal cardiac irregularity, caused by continuous interplay of the parasympathetic and sympathetic nervous systems

CLINICAL
ALERT

   2. Long-term variability: rhythmic fluctuations and waves; usually occur three to five times/minute
   3. Short-term variability: the beat-to-beat changes of heart rate in the baseline; average beat-to-beat variability is 6 to 10 beats/minute
   4. Increased variability
      a. Cause: early, mild hypoxia and fetal stimulation
      b. Clinical significance: earliest sign of mild fetal hypoxia
      c. Nursing interventions: carefully evaluate the FHR tracing for signs of fetal distress
   5. Decreased variability
      a. Cause: hypoxia, acidosis, central nervous system depressants, medications
      b. Clinical significance: benign when associated with drugs; ominous if caused by hypoxia or associated with late decelerations
      c. Nursing interventions: assist with possible fetal blood sampling and insertion of internal monitor, as ordered

D. Diagnostic measures
   1. Fetal blood sampling
      a. Definition: method of monitoring fetal blood pH when indefinite or nonreassuring FHR patterns occur
      b. Procedure: sample is usually taken from the scalp but also may be taken from the presenting part if the fetus is in a breech presentation
      c. Requirements: membranes must be ruptured, the cervix must be dilated at least 2 to 3 cm, and the presenting part must be no higher than -2 station
      d. Results: 7.25 and higher is normal, 7.20 to 7.24 is preacidotic, and lower than 7.2 constitutes severe acidosis
   2. Amnioinfusion
      a. Definition: replacement of amniotic fluid volume through intrauterine infusion of a saline solution using a pressure catheter
      b. Indications: repetitive variable decelerations not alleviated by maternal position change and oxygen administration
      c. Benefits: relieves umbilical cord compression in such conditions as oligohydramnios associated with postmaturity, intrauterine growth retardation, and premature rupture of membranes

♦ XI. Obstetric procedures

A. Episiotomy: incision of the perineum to enlarge the vaginal outlet
   1. Type: depends on the site and direction of the incision
   2. Advantages
      a. Prevents tearing (laceration) of the perineum
      b. Can be repaired more easily than a tear and heals faster

      c. Enlarges the vaginal outlet to facilitate manipulation or use of forceps

   3. Disadvantages

      a. May interfere with maternal-neonatal bonding if discomfort is severe

      b. Creates a potential site of infection

      c. May make the patient hesitant to void or have a bowel movement

B. Forceps delivery

   1. Commonly used forceps: Kjelland, Elliot, Piper, Tucker-McLean, and Simpson

   2. Types of delivery

      a. Outlet (low) forceps: when the fetus's head is visible on the perineum

      b. Midforceps: when the head is located at the ischial spines (rarely performed)

   3. Advantage: shortens the second stage of labor when adverse fetal and maternal conditions exist

   4. Disadvantages

      a. Increases perinatal morbidity and mortality (midforceps delivery)

      b. Increases neonatal birth trauma and depression

      c. Increases incidence of postpartum hemorrhage

C. Vacuum extraction

   1. Alternative to forceps to facilitate descent of fetal head

   2. After a plastic vacuum cup is applied to the fetal head, negative pressure is exerted and traction is applied to deliver the head

   3. Advantages

      a. Lower incidence of vaginal, cervical, and third- and fourth- degree lacerations

      b. Less maternal discomfort, since the cup does not occupy additional space in the birth canal

   4. Disadvantages

      a. Marked caput succedaneum possible as long as 7 days after birth

      b. Tentorial tears possible from extreme pressure

D. Cesarean delivery: removal of the infant from the uterus through an abdominal incision

   1. Indications

      a. Cephalopelvic disproportion

      b. Uterine dysfunction

      c. Malposition or malpresentation

      d. Previous uterine surgery

      e. Complete or partial placenta previa

      f. Preexisting medical condition (for example, diabetes or cardiac disease)

g. Prolapsed umbilical cord

h. Fetal distress

2. Uterine incisions

a. Transverse

(1) Preferred and most common incision

(2) Decreased incidence of peritonitis and postoperative adhesions

(3) Minimal loss of blood

b. Classic (vertical); used when adhesions from previous cesarean exist, when the fetus is in a transverse lie, and with an anteriorly implanted placenta

E. Vaginal birth after previous cesarean delivery (VBAC)

1. A patient who had a previous low transverse cesarean delivery may attempt a vaginal birth provided there is no medical or obstetric contraindication to labor and no history of prior uterine rupture

2. The incidence of dehiscence of a former low transverse uterine incision dehiscence during an attempted VBAC is less than 1%

♦ XII. Induction of labor

A. General information

1. Factors that determine readiness for induction

a. Fetal maturity (assessed by amniotic fluid studies and serial ultrasound examinations)

b. Fetal position (determined by ultrasound or Leopold's maneuvers)

c. Cervical dilation, effacement, consistency, and position (determined by vaginal examination and use of scoring systems, such as BISHOP SCORE)

2. Indications for induction

a. Postmaturity (greater than 42 weeks of gestation), which can lead to placental insufficiency or fetal compromise

b. Premature rupture of membranes, which increases the risk of intrauterine infection

c. Pregnancy-induced hypertension, which may worsen

d. Rh isoimmunization, which can produce erythroblastosis fetalis

e. Maternal diabetes, which can lead to fetal death from placental insufficiency

f. Fetal death

3. Maternal contraindications for induction

a. Grand multiparity

b. Placental abnormalities

c. Previous uterine surgery

d. Overdistention of the uterus

e. Structural abnormalities of the vagina, uterus, or pelvis

TEACHING TIPS
Patient receiving labor induction

Be sure to include the following topics in your teaching plan for the patient receiving induction:
- Rationale for induction
- Type of induction being used
- Possible risks and benefits to patient and fetus
- Signs and symptoms to report
- Necessary assessments and monitoring activities to be performed

4. Fetal contraindications for induction
   a. Abnormal fetal lie
   b. Fetal distress
   c. Premature or low-birth-weight fetus
   d. Positive oxytocin challenge test
5. Advantages of induction
   a. Allows the patient to prepare physically and psychologically for labor and delivery
   b. Can resolve medical conditions that might endanger fetal well-being
6. Disadvantages of induction
   a. Poses risks to the fetus from increased uterine activity and possible prematurity
   b. Poses risks to the patient from prolonged labor, cervical laceration, and postpartum hemorrhage
   c. Produces physical and psychological stress if induction fails

B. Induction by way of amniotomy: artificial rupturing of membranes with a sterile instrument; under favorable conditions, approximately 80% of patients will enter labor within 24 hours
   1. Advantages
      a. Facilitates fetal status monitoring using an internal scalp electrode, catheter, or scalp blood sampling
      b. Facilitates assessment of amniotic fluid color and composition
   2. Disadvantages
      a. Increases the risk of infection and cord prolapse
      b. Increases the incidence of fetal head compression
   3. Indications
      a. When internal fetal monitoring is desired
      b. When oxytocin is contraindicated

   4. Contraindications
      a. Presenting part at -2 station or higher
      b. Placenta previa
      c. Abnormal presenting part
      d. Uncertain estimated date of delivery
      e. Active herpesvirus II lesions in the vagina

C. Induction by way of oxytocin infusion: administration of intravenous oxytocin (Pitocin) to augment or stimulate uterine contractions
   1. Advantages
      a. Uses a drug with a predictable action
      b. Does not directly affect the fetus
      c. Stimulates contractions efficiently and effectively
   2. Disadvantage: increases the risk of tetanic uterine contractions and overstimulation of the uterus, which can lead to fetal distress and uterine rupture
   3. Indications
      a. Prolonged rupture of membranes
      b. Postmaturity
      c. Induction necessary because of adverse maternal or fetal conditions
   4. Contraindications
      a. Cephalopelvic disproportion
      b. Fetal distress
      c. Previous uterine surgery
      d. Overdistended uterus
      e. Abnormal fetal presentation
   5. Nursing interventions

CLINICAL ALERT

      a. Assess the FHR and contraction patterns by continuous electronic monitoring
      b. Stop the infusion immediately if fetal distress or tetanic uterine contractions occur
      c. Continue interventions discussed in Section VI of this chapter

D. Induction using prostaglandin gel: intracervical or intravaginal insertion of prostaglandin gel to soften the cervix
   1. Advantages
      a. Decreases the likelihood of cesarean delivery or failed induction
      b. Requires lower doses of oxytocin
      c. Reduces the need for analgesia or such instruments as forceps
      d. Shortens labor
   2. Disadvantage: increases the risk of uterine hyperstimulation

3. Indications
   a. Postmaturity
   b. Long, thick cervix at the time of induction
   c. Induction necessary because of adverse maternal or fetal conditions
4. Contraindications
   a. Maternal temperature greater than 100° F (37.8° C)
   b. Asthma or cardiac disorder
   c. Vaginal bleeding
   d. Allergy to prostaglandin
   e. Bishop score higher than 5
5. Nursing considerations
   a. The procedure is not approved by the Food and Drug Administration for cervical softening
   b. Additional cervical softening is unlikely to result from additional doses when the Bishop score is 7 or higher
   c. The patient should remain recumbent for at least 15 minutes after gel insertion

CLINICAL ALERT

   d. The nurse should perform continuous external fetal monitoring for 4 hours after gel insertion

◆ XIII. Obstetrical analgesia and anesthesia

A. Pain perception
   1. Theories of pain
      a. Specificity: a specific pain system carries messages from pain receptors in the body to a pain center in the brain
      b. Pattern: particular networks of nerve impulses are produced by sensory input at the dorsal horn cells; pain results when the output of these cells exceeds a critical level
      c. Gate control: local physical stimulation can balance the pain stimuli by closing down a hypothetical gate in the spinal cord that blocks pain signals from reaching the brain

B. Sources of pain during labor
   1. Dilation and stretching of the cervix
   2. Hypoxia of the uterine muscle cells during a contraction
   3. Lower uterine segment stretching
   4. Pressure by the presenting part on adjacent structures
   5. Distention of the vagina and perineum
   6. Emotional tension

C. Factors affecting pain perception
1. Cultural background: individuals tend to react to pain in ways that are acceptable in that culture
2. Personal significance: self-concept is closely aligned with how an individual regards pain
3. Fatigue and sleep deprivation: a tired individual has less energy and cannot focus on such strategies as distraction
4. Attention and distractions: preoccupation with another activity (such as breathing techniques) lessens pain perception

◆ XIV. Pain relief during labor and delivery

A. Nonpharmacologic measures
1. Effleurage: light abdominal stroking with the fingertips in a circular motion; effective for mild to moderate discomfort
2. Distraction: diversion of attention from discomfort during early labor (for example, by playing games or recalling pleasant experiences)
3. Lamaze breathing: three patterns of controlled chest breathing, used primarily during the active and transitional phases of labor
   a. Slow: inhaling through the nose and exhaling through the mouth or nose six to nine times/minute
   b. Accelerated-decelerated: inhaling through the nose and exhaling through the mouth as contractions become more intense
   c. Pant-blow: rapid, shallow breathing through the mouth only throughout contractions, particularly during the transitional phase
4. Transcutaneous electrical nerve stimulation: stimulation of large-diameter neural fibers using electric currents to alter pain perception
5. Hypnosis: altered state of consciousness allowing perception and motor control to be influenced by suggestion
6. Acupuncture and acupressure: stimulation of key trigger points with needles (acupuncture) or finger pressure (acupressure) in order to reduce pain and enhance energy flow

B. ANALGESIC agents
1. Opiates
   a. A commonly used drug is meperidine (Demerol)
   b. Common maternal adverse reactions are respiratory depression, nausea and vomiting, drowsiness, and transient hypotension
   c. Common fetal-neonatal adverse reactions include neonatal respiratory depression (if medication is given within 2 hours of delivery), hypotonia, and lethargy
2. Sedatives
   a. Barbiturates, such as secobarbital (Seconal) and pentobarbital sodium (Nembutal), are sometimes used in false labor or in the early latent phase of labor

    b. Some doctors may use benzodiazepines, such as midazolam (Versed)

C. ANESTHETIC agents

  1. GENERAL ANESTHESIA: administered I.V. or by inhalation, resulting in unconsciousness; used only if regional anesthesia is contraindicated or in a rapidly developing emergency

    a. Inhalation anesthetics: nitrous oxide, isoflurane (Forane), and halothane (Fluothane)

    b. I.V. anesthetics (usually reserved for patients with massive blood loss): thiopental (Pentothal), and ketamine (Ketalar)

    c. Maternal adverse reactions: vomiting and aspiration; increased uterine relaxation, possibly leading to postpartum uterine atony

    d. Fetal-neonatal adverse reactions: respiratory depression, fetal acidosis, hypotonia, and lethargy

  2. REGIONAL ANESTHESIA: LOCAL ANESTHESIA administered to block pain neuropathways that pass from the uterus to the spinal cord by way of sympathetic nerves

    a. Lumbar epidural anesthesia: injection of medication into the epidural space in the lumbar region

      (1) Advantages

        (a) Leaves the patient awake and cooperative

        (b) Provides analgesia for the first and second stages and anesthesia for delivery without adverse fetal effects

      (2) Disadvantages

        (a) Hypotension (uncommon, although incidence increases if the patient does not receive a proper fluid load before the procedure)

        (b) Decreased urge to push (uncommon because of the low concentration of local anesthetic used)

        (c) Risk of dural puncture, leading to postspinal headache or transient complete motor paralysis

    b. Spinal anesthesia: injection of medication into the cerebrospinal fluid in the spinal canal

      (1) Advantages

        (a) Low incidence of adverse effects

        (b) Useful for urgent cesarean sections because of its rapid onset

      (2) Disadvantages

        (a) Short duration

        (b) Postspinal headache

        (c) Risk of transient complete motor paralysis

        (d) Increased incidence and degree of hypotension

        (e) Urine retention

  c. Local infiltration: injection of anesthesia into the perineal nerves
   (1) Advantage: ease of administration
   (2) Disadvantage: no relief from discomfort during labor, only at delivery
  d. Pudendal block: blockage of the pudendal nerve (used only for delivery, not for labor)
   (1) Advantage: a simple, safe method that usually does not depress the fetus
   (2) Disadvantage: no relief from discomfort of uterine contractions, only discomfort from perineal distention
  e. Paracervical block: blockage of nerves in the peridural space at the sacral hiatus
   (1) Advantages
    (a) Patient is awake
    (b) Provides analgesia for the first and second stages of labor
    (c) Provides anesthesia for delivery
   (2) Disadvantages
    (a) Increased incidence of hypotension
    (b) Increased use of forceps
    (c) Increased fetal bradycardia
    (d) Increased risk of hematomas
    (e) Risk of injecting directly into the fetus

D. Nursing interventions
 1. Know each type of anesthesia and analgesia used in obstetrics
 2. Allay the patient's fears and anxieties about medication, and answer the patient's questions

 3. Help the anesthesiologist and obstetrician
 4. Closely monitor patient and fetus; watch for possible maternal, fetal, or neonatal complications from medications administered
 5. Take swift action if adverse reactions occur

♦ XV. Optional birthing experiences

A. Birth centers
 1. Birth centers may be found in maternity facilities located in a hospital or separate institution close to a hospital
 2. Centers provide a warm, home-like environment
 3. Families are required to take more responsibility for the birth experience
 4. Centers are not appropriate for high-risk deliveries
 5. Most care is provided by nurse-midwives

B. Home births: controversial option because of inadequate medical backup

C. Siblings present at birth: prenatal education of and active participation by siblings foster the integration of the neonate into the family

D. Optional positioning: alternatives to the lithotomy position include side-lying, squatting, sitting, and semi-Fowler's positions

E. Leboyer method: controversial, soothing, tender approach to handling the neonate immediately after delivery
1. Lights are dimmed
2. Noise is diminished
3. The neonate is gently placed in a warm bath after the umbilical cord has been clamped

♦ XVI. Role of the coach during labor and delivery

A. Coach
1. A coach is of great value during labor and delivery, especially if the patient and coach have attended prenatal classes together
2. The coach may be the patient's husband or any significant other
3. The patient's coach can provide several benefits

B. Benefits
1. Emotional support
2. Physical support (such as back rubs)
3. Enhanced communication between the patient and staff, if necessary (for example, to overcome a language barrier)
4. Reduction in anxiety and pain perception
5. Aid in the initiation of bonding with the neonate

POINTS TO REMEMBER

♦ Many theories on labor initiation have been proposed, but none has been proven.

♦ The three major components of labor are the passage, passenger, and power.

♦ Labor is divided into four stages.

♦ A contraction's duration is measured from the beginning of one contraction to the end of that contraction; frequency is measured from the beginning of one contraction to the beginning of the next one.

♦ The patient's understanding of the potential sources of pain during labor and delivery may help alleviate anxiety.

◆ Pain perception is an individualized reaction that is influenced by physical, sociocultural, and psychological factors.

◆ The nurse must be familiar enough with anesthetic and analgesic agents to answer a patient's questions, assist the anesthesiologist and obstetrician, and identify adverse maternal, fetal, and neonatal effects quickly.

◆ The patient's blood pressure must be monitored after epidural, spinal, and paracervical regional anesthesia.

STUDY QUESTIONS

To evaluate your understanding of this chapter, answer the following questions in the space provided; then compare your responses with the correct answers in Appendix B, pages 173 and 174.

1. Which physiologic events and maternal behaviors characterize the active phase of the first stage of labor?_____

_____

_____

2. What is the primary activity during the fourth stage of labor? _____

_____

_____

3. How should the nurse intervene if the patient's blood pressure drops during labor or delivery? _____

_____

_____

4. What are the six mechanisms of labor? _____

_____

_____

5. Which fetal characteristics affect labor?_____

_____

_____

6. How does the maternal respiratory system respond during labor?_____

_____

_____

7. What are three advantages of external electronic fetal monitoring? _____

_____

_____

8. What are the three phases of a uterine contraction? _____

_____

_____

9. What causes variable decelerations of fetal heart rate? _____

_____

_____

10. When is a cesarean delivery indicated? _____

_____

_____

11. Readiness for induction depends on which factors? _____

_____

_____

12. What methods can be used to induce labor? _____

_____

_____

CRITICAL THINKING AND APPLICATION EXERCISES

1. Develop a table comparing the physiologic and psychosocial events associated with each stage of labor.

2. Create a patient-specific instruction sheet about the signs of true labor.

3. Review copies of uterine monitoring and fetal heart rate tracings. Identify the phases of the uterine contraction and fetal heart rate pattern seen.

4. Follow a patient admitted in labor through delivery of the neonate. Develop a patient-specific plan of care including any physiologic and psychosocial needs.

CHAPTER

7

Complications and High-Risk Conditions of Labor and Delivery

LEARNING OBJECTIVES

After studying this chapter, you should be able to:

♦ List possible complications of labor and delivery.

♦ Describe management of the patient in premature labor.

♦ Describe immediate steps to follow when an umbilical cord prolapses.

CHAPTER OVERVIEW

During labor and delivery, conditions may develop that cause complications or place the patient at risk. Throughout this period, the nurse must be alert for these conditions to ensure early identification and prompt intervention, thereby minimizing the risk to the patient and fetus.

◆ I. Possible complications

A. DYSTOCIA: difficult labor

1. Mechanical causes: contracted pelvis and obstructive tumors (maternal); malpresentation or malformation (fetal)
2. Functional causes: hypertonic or hypotonic uterine patterns

B. Premature rupture of membranes: rupture one or more hours before the onset of labor

1. Associated findings: malpresentation, incompetent cervix, subclinical infection, multiparity, and preterm labor
2. Maternal-fetal implications: chorioamnionitis if the latent period (time between rupture of membranes and onset of labor) is longer than 24 hours; signs include fetal tachycardia, maternal fever, foul-smelling amniotic fluid, and uterine tenderness
3. Fetal-neonatal implications: increased incidence of fetal infection and perinatal mortality
4. Management
   a. Antibiotic administration, if indicated
   b. Assessment for signs of infection or fetal distress
   c. Possible induction of labor or cesarean delivery if labor does not start within 24 hours

C. Precipitate labor: labor that lasts three hours or less, usually caused by lack of maternal tissue resistance to the passage of the fetus

D. Amniotic fluid embolism: escape of amniotic fluid into the maternal circulation resulting from a defect in the membranes after rupture or from partial abruptio placentae

1. Fetal-neonatal implications: possible deposition of meconium, lanugo, and vernix in the pulmonary arterioles
2. Clinical manifestations: sudden dyspnea, cyanosis, tachypnea, hemorrhage, chest pain, coughing with pink frothy sputum, increasing restlessness and anxiety, and shock disproportionate to blood loss
3. Predisposing factors: intrauterine fetal death, high parity, abruptio placentae, oxytocin augmentation, advanced maternal age
4. Management
   a. Administration of oxygen, blood, and heparin
   b. Insertion of a central venous pressure line
   c. Monitoring of cardiopulmonary status
   d. Immediate delivery of the infant

E. Prolapsed umbilical cord: descent of the umbilical cord into the vagina before the presenting part

1. Fetal-neonatal implications

CLINICAL
ALERT

a. The cord may become compressed between the fetus and maternal cervix or pelvis, thus compromising fetoplacental perfusion

b. Umbilical cord prolapse is an emergency requiring prompt action to save the fetus

2. Predisposing factors: abnormal fetal position, multiple gestation, hydramnios, rupture of membranes before engagement, and factors that could interfere with fetal descent

CLINICAL
ALERT

3. Management

a. Use of Trendelenburg or knee-chest position to cause fetal head to fall back from cord

b. FHR monitoring with observation for decelerations

c. Application of saline-soaked sterile dressing over any portion of the cord if exposed

d. Pushing of the head up and off the cord with a sterile gloved hand

e. Immediate delivery

F. Inverted uterus: partial or total inversion of the uterus during delivery of the placenta

1. Causes

a. Excessive traction on the umbilical cord

b. Thin uterine wall

2. Clinical manifestations: severe uterine pain, hemorrhage, inability to palpate the fundus abdominally, and uterine mass within the vaginal canal

3. Management

a. Administration of fluids, blood, and oxygen

b. Monitoring of vital signs

c. Immediate manual replacement by the doctor

d. Possible emergency hysterectomy

G. Early postpartum hemorrhage: blood loss of 500 ml or more during the first hour after delivery

1. Causes

a. Uterine atony (accounts for 80% to 90% of all early hemorrhages)

b. Lacerations of the vagina and cervix

c. Hematoma formation

2. Management

a. Assessment of post-delivery uterine contractions, amount and color of vaginal bleeding, presence of distended bladder, and vital signs every 15 minutes until stable

b. I.V. administration of oxytocin

c. Vaginal examination for possible bleeding sites

d. Uterine massage

3. Risk factors
   a. Delivery of a large neonate or multiple births
   b. General anesthesia
   c. Labor augmented with oxytocin
   d. Forceps delivery or rotation
   e. High parity or previous history of hemorrhage
   f. Vaginal birth after previous cesarean delivery

H. Fetal distress: fetal compromise that results in a stressful and potentially lethal condition
   1. Causes
      a. Prematurity
      b. Uteroplacental insufficiency
      c. Congenital malformation
      d. ABO or Rh incompatibility
      e. Maternal complications, such as diabetes, heart disease, or pregnancy-induced hypertension
      f. Long labor
      g. Postmaturity
      h. Oxytocin infusion
      i. Vaginal bleeding
   2. Management
      a. Monitor the FHR, fetal activity, fetal heart variability
      b. Notify the doctor immediately
      c. Prepare for possible placement of internal monitor and fetal scalp pH sampling
      d. Position the patient on her left side
      e. Administer oxygen via face mask according to hospital protocol or the doctor's orders (typically 6 to 8 liters/minute)
      f. Discontinue oxytocin infusion

I. Lacerations: tears in the perineum, vagina, or cervix from stretching of tissues during delivery; perineal lacerations are classified as first, second, third, and fourth degree
   1. First-degree laceration: involving the vaginal mucosa and the skin of the perineum to the fourchette
   2. Second-degree laceration: involving the vagina, perineal skin, fascia, levator ani muscle, and perineal body
   3. Third-degree laceration: involving the entire perineum and the external anal sphincter
   4. Fourth-degree laceration: involving the entire perineum, rectal sphincter, and portions of the rectal mucous membrane

J. Disseminated intravascular coagulation: increased production of prothrombin, platelets, and other coagulation factors that leads to widespread thrombi formation, depletion of clotting factors, and hemorrhage

1. Predisposing factors: abruptio placentae, sepsis, intrauterine fetal death, and amniotic fluid embolism
2. Clinical manifestations: thrombocytopenia, decreased fibrinogen level and platelet count, increased prothrombin time, and partial thromboplastin time
3. Maternal implication: death if hypofibrinogenemia does not reverse
4. Fetal-neonatal implications: major risk of hypoxia; also at risk from maternal sepsis, acidosis, and hypotension
5. Management
   a. Blood and fibrinogen transfusions
   b. Treatment of underlying condition
   c. Administration of heparin
   d. Immediate delivery

K. HELLP syndrome: hypertensive state in pregnancy that includes Hemolysis of red blood cells, Elevated Liver enzymes, and Low Platelets, in addition to the typical criteria for severe preeclampsia

1. Clinical manifestations
   a. Anemia, fatigue, pallor, anorexia, dyspnea, and edema caused by hemolysis of red blood cells
   b. Thrombocytopenia (less than $100,000/\mu l$)
2. Management
   a. Maintain adequate fluid volume
   b. Prevent hemorrhage
   c. Monitor liver function
   d. Prevent fetal hypoxia

◆ II. Premature labor

A. Definition: labor that occurs before the end of the 37th week of pregnancy; places patient and fetus at high risk

B. Maternal causes
1. Cardiovascular and renal disease
2. Diabetes mellitus
3. Pregnancy-induced hypertension
4. Infection
5. Abdominal surgery or trauma
6. Incompetent cervix
7. Placental abnormalities
8. Premature rupture of membranes

C. Fetal causes
   1. Infection
   2. Hydramnios
   3. Multiple pregnancy

D. Fetal-neonatal implications: increased risk of morbidity or mortality from excessive maturational deficiencies (see Chapter 5, XIV)

E. Management with commonly used TOCOLYTIC AGENTS
   1. Terbutaline sulfate (Brethine) and Ritodrine (Yutopar)
      a. Mechanism: beta$_2$ receptor stimulation, causing smooth muscle relaxation
      b. Contraindications
         (1) Gestation less than 20 weeks
         (2) Cervical dilation greater than 4 cm
         (3) Cervical effacement greater than 50%
         (4) Severe pregnancy-induced hypertension
         (5) Cardiac disease
      c. Maternal adverse effects: tachycardia, diarrhea, nervousness and tremors, nausea and vomiting, headache, hyperglycemia or hypoglycemia, hypokalemia, pulmonary edema
      d. Fetal adverse effects: tachycardia, hypoxia, hypoglycemia, and hypocalcemia
      e. Antidote: propranolol (Inderal)
   2. Magnesium sulfate
      a. Mechanism: reflux of calcium into the myometrial cells is prevented, thus maintaining a relaxed uterus
      b. Adverse effects: toxicity is manifested by central nervous system depression in the mother
   3. Indomethacin (Indocin)
      a. Mechanism: nonsteroidal anti-inflammatory agent that decreases production of prostaglandins, lipid compounds associated with the initiation of labor
      b. Adverse effects

CLINICAL ALERT

         (1) Maternal symptoms (nausea, vomiting, and dyspepsia)
         (2) Should not be used after 32 weeks' gestation in order to avoid premature closure of the ductus arteriosus
   4. Nifedipine (Procardia)
      a. Mechanism: calcium channel blocker that decreases production of calcium, a substance associated with the initiation of labor
      b. Adverse effects: dizziness, nausea, bradycardia, flushing

F. Nursing interventions
   1. Provide emotional support
   2. Monitor laboratory results
   3. Monitor maternal vital signs and FHR

TEACHING TIPS
Patient receiving home tocolytic therapy

Be sure to include the following topics in your teaching plan for the patient who will be receiving home tocolytic therapy:
- Rationale for therapy
- Drug dosage, frequency and route
- Possible adverse effects
- Signs and symptoms of true labor
- Daily fetal movement counts
- Contraction and pulse rate monitoring
- Signs and symptoms to notify doctor
- Activity restrictions
- Supportive services

CLINICAL ALERT

4. Monitor status of contractions
5. Notify the doctor if the maternal pulse rate exceeds 120 beats/minute or the FHR exceeds 180 beats/minute
6. Place the patient in the lateral position to increase placental perfusion
7. Have antidotes readily available
8. If appropriate, allow patient to be discharged home on tocolytic therapy with home nursing care follow-up

POINTS TO REMEMBER

♦ An umbilical cord prolapse requires immediate intervention to save the fetus.

♦ An early postpartum hemorrhage occurs when a patient loses at least 500 ml of blood in the first hour after delivery.

♦ Uterine atony causes most early postpartum hemorrhages.

♦ Lacerations are classified as first-, second-, third-, or fourth-degree lacerations.

♦ HELLP syndrome refers to the hypertensive condition in pregnancy that is characterized by Hemolysis of red blood cells, Elevated Liver enzymes, and Low Platelets.

STUDY QUESTIONS

To evaluate your understanding of this chapter, answer the following questions in the space provided; then compare your responses with the correct answers in Appendix B, page 174.

1. What do the letters in HELLP syndrome signify? _____

   _____

   _____

2. How do terbutaline, magnesium sulfate, indomethacin, and nifedipine stop contractions?_____

   _____

   _____

3. What does management of the woman with a postpartum hemorrhage include? _____

   _____

   _____

4. What are the potential maternal-fetal implications of premature rupture of membranes? _____

   _____

   _____

CRITICAL THINKING AND APPLICATION EXERCISES

1. Interview a patient who has experienced a complication during labor and delivery. Prepare an oral presentation for your fellow classmates detailing the patient's experiences and what was done.

2. Develop a patient instruction sheet for the patient with premature rupture of membranes.

3. Follow a patient with a complication of labor and delivery through the labor and delivery period. Develop a patient-specific plan of care including any needs for education and supportive measures.

CHAPTER

The Normal Neonate

LEARNING OBJECTIVES

After studying this chapter, you should be able to:

◆ Explain how to perform neonatal care.

◆ Describe the normal physical and neurologic characteristics of the neonate.

◆ Name at least five factors to include in a gestational age assessment.

◆ State the advantages and disadvantages of breast-feeding and bottle-feeding.

CHAPTER OVERVIEW

A newborn experiences many changes while adapting to extrauterine existence. Knowledge of these changes and of the normal physical and neurologic characteristics of the NEONATE provides the basis for normal newborn care.

◆ I. Adaptation to extrauterine life

A. Cardiovascular system

    1. The first breath expands the neonate's lungs, decreasing pulmonary vascular resistance

    2. Clamping the cord increases systemic vascular resistance and left atrial pressure

    3. Major changes occur as the neonate adapts to extrauterine life

       a. Changing atrial pressures functionally close the foramen ovale (fibrosis may take from several weeks to a year)

       b. Increasing P_{O_2} constricts the ductus arteriosus

         (1) Functional closure occurs within 15 minutes after birth; fibrosis within 3 weeks

         (2) The ductus arteriosus eventually occludes and becomes a ligament

       c. Clamping and severing of the umbilical cord immediately closes the umbilical vein, arteries, and ductus venosus (fibrosis occurs within 3 to 7 days, and the structures eventually convert into ligaments)

B. Respiratory system

    1. The initial breath is a reflex triggered in response to chilling, noise, light, or pressure changes

    2. Air replaces the fluid that filled the lungs before birth

       a. Approximately 7 to 42 ml of amniotic fluid is squeezed or drained from the lungs during vaginal delivery; other lung fluid crosses the alveolar membrane into the capillaries

       b. Fluid retention greatly impedes normal respiratory adjustment

C. Renal system

    1. Renal function does not fully mature until after the first year of life; as a result, the neonate has a minimal range of chemical balance and safety

    2. Low ability to excrete drugs and excessive fluid loss can rapidly lead to acidosis and fluid imbalances

D. Gastrointestinal system

    1. Bacteria are not normally present in the neonate's gastrointestinal tract

    2. Bowel sounds can be heard one hour after birth

    3. Uncoordinated peristaltic activity in the esophagus exists for the first few days of life

    4. The neonate has a limited ability to digest fats because amylase and lipase are absent at birth

5. The lower intestine contains meconium at birth; the first meconium (sterile, greenish black, and viscous) usually passes within 24 hours

E. Thermogenesis
   1. Normal neonates can produce sufficient heat in an optimal thermal environment
   2. Rapid heat loss may occur in a suboptimal thermal environment via CONDUCTION, CONVECTION, RADIATION, or EVAPORATION

F. Immunologic system
   1. IgG, a placentally transferred immunoglobin, provides the neonate with antibodies to bacterial and viral agents
     a. IgG can be detected in the fetus at the 3rd month of gestation
     b. The infant first synthesizes its own IgG during the first 3 months of life, thus compensating for concurrent catabolism of maternal antibodies
   2. The fetus synthesizes IgM by the 20th week of gestation
     a. IgM does not cross the placenta
     b. High levels of IgM in the neonate indicate a nonspecific infection
   3. IgA is not detectable at birth; it does not cross the placenta
     a. Secretory IgA is found in colostrum and breast milk
     b. IgA limits bacterial growth in the gastrointestinal tract

G. Hematopoietic system: blood volume of the full-term neonate is approximately 80 to 85 ml/kg of body weight (for additional information, see Appendix D: Normal Neonatal Laboratory Values, page 178)

H. Neurologic system (see Section III, P in this chapter)

I. Hepatic system
   1. *Physiologic jaundice* (icterus neonatorum) develops in about 50% of full-term neonates and 80% of premature neonates
     a. The icteric (yellow) color reflects increased serum levels of unconjugated bilirubin from increased red blood cell lysis, altered bilirubin conjugation, or increased bilirubin reabsorption from the gastrointestinal tract
     b. The icteric color is not apparent until the bilirubin levels are approximately 4 to 6 mg/dl
     c. Unconjugated bilirubin levels seldom exceed 12 mg/dl; peak levels occur by 3 to 5 days after delivery (full-term) and 5 to 6 days (preterm)
     d. Physiologic jaundice appears after the first 24 hours of extrauterine life; pathologic jaundice is evident at birth or within the first 24 hours of extrauterine life (see Chapter 9, Section V)
   2. *Breast milk jaundice* appears after the first week of extrauterine life when physiologic jaundice is declining

   a. Peak level is 15 to 25 mg/dl

   b. About 1% to 2% of breast-feeding neonates are affected

   c. Its exact cause is unknown; current theories revolve around increased intestinal absorption of bilirubin from beta-glucuronidase

  3. *Breast-feeding-associated jaundice* appears on the second or third day of extrauterine life in about 10% of breast-fed neonates

   a. Peak level is 9.0 to 19.0 mg/dl

   b. Poor caloric intake leads to decreased hepatic transport and bilirubin clearance

  4. Management of jaundice includes monitoring serum bilirubin levels, maintaining hydration, using bilirubin lights as needed, and providing emotional support to the parents

♦ II. Neonatal assessment

A. Initial assessment

  1. Ensure a proper airway via suctioning; administer oxygen as needed

  2. Dry the neonate under the warmer; keep the head lower than the trunk to promote drainage of secretions

  3. Apply a cord clamp, and monitor the neonate for abnormal bleeding from the cord

  4. Observe the neonate for voiding and meconium

  5. Assess the neonate for gross abnormalities and clinical manifestations of suspected abnormalities

  6. Continue to assess the neonate by using the Apgar score criteria even after the 5-minute score is received (see *Apgar score*)

  7. Obtain clear footprints and fingerprints (the neonate's footprints are kept on a record that includes the mother's fingerprint)

  8. Apply identification bands with matching numbers to the mother (one band) and neonate (two bands) before they leave the delivery room

  9. Promote bonding between the mother and neonate

B. Ongoing physical assessments

  1. Assess the neonate's vital signs

   a. Take the first temperature rectally to check for rectal patency

    (1) Continued use of the rectal site is not recommended because of possible rectal mucosa damage

    (2) A delay in adjusting to extrauterine existence may cause temperature at birth to be 96.8° F (36° C), but this should stabilize within 8 to 12 hours at approximately 98.2° F (36.8° C)

   b. Take the apical pulse for 60 seconds (normal rate is 120 to 160 beats/minute)

Apgar score

The Apgar score is a five-part scoring method used to evaluate the neonate at 1 and 5 minutes after birth. A score of 8 to 10 indicates that the neonate is in no apparent distress; a score below 8 indicates that resuscitative measures may be needed.

SIGN	0	1	2
Heart rate	Absent	Less than 100 beats/minute	Greater than 100 beats/minute
Respiratory effort	Absent	Slow, irregular	Good crying
Muscle tone	Flaccid	Some flexion of extremities	Active motion
Reflex irritability	None	Grimace	Vigorous cry
Color	Pale, blue	Body pink, blue extremities	Completely pink

    c. Count respirations with a stethoscope for 60 seconds (normal rate is 30 to 60 breaths/minute)

    d. Measure and record blood pressure (normal reading ranges from 60/40 mm Hg to 90/45 mm Hg)

  2. Measure and record the neonate's vital statistics

    a. Average weight is 6½ to 7¾ lb (2,950 to 3,515 g)

    b. Average length is 18″ to 20½″ (45.7 to 52.1 cm)

    c. Average head circumference is 13″ to 14″ (33 to 35 cm)

    d. Average chest circumference is 12½″ (32 cm)

  3. Complete a gestational age assessment if indicated (see *Ballard gestational-age assessment tool,* pages 104 and 105)

C. Administer prescribed medications

  1. Vitamin K (AquaMEPHYTON) is administered prophylactically to prevent a transient deficiency of coagulation factors II, VII, IX, and X

  2. Erythromycin ointment (Ilotycin) is the drug of choice for prophylactic eye treatment of *Neisseria gonorrhoeae* and *Chlamydia;* treatment is legally required

D. Perform laboratory tests

  1. Monitor hematocrit and glucose levels

  2. Test results aid in assessing for anemia and hypoglycemia

Text continues on page 107.

Ballard gestational-age assessment tool

To use this tool, the examiner evaluates and scores the neuromuscular and physical maturity criteria, totals the scores, then plots the sum in the maturity rating box to determine gestational age. Unlike portions of the Dubowitz neurologic examination, the Ballard neuromuscular examination can be done even if the neonate is not alert.

NEUROMUSCULAR MATURITY

Neuromuscular Maturity Sign	Score							Record Score Here
	-1	0	1	2	3	4	5	
Posture	–						–	
Square window (wrist)	>90°	90°	60°	45°	30°	0°	–	
Arm recoil	–	180°	140° to 180°	110° to 140°	90° to 110°	<90°	–	
Popliteal angle	180°	160°	140°	120°	100°	90°	<90°	
Scarf sign							–	
Heel to ear							–	
					Total neuromuscular maturity score			

PHYSICAL MATURITY

Physical Maturity Sign	Score							Record Score Here
	-1	0	1	2	3	4	5	
Posture	Sticky, friable, transparent	Gelatinous, red, translucent	Smooth, pink, visible vessels	Superficial peeling or rash; few visible vessels	Cracking: pale areas; rare visible vessels	Parchment-like; deep cracking; no visible vessels	Leathery, cracked, wrinkled	
Lanugo	None	Sparse	Abundant	Thinning	Bald areas	Mostly bald	–	

Ballard gestational-age assessment tool (continued)

Physical Maturity Sign	Score							Record Score Here
	-1	0	1	2	3	4	5	
Plantar surface	Heel-toe 40 to 50 mm; -1; <40 mm: -2	<50 mm; no crease	Faint red marks	Anterior transverse crease only	Creases over anterior two-thirds	Creases over entire sole	–	
Breast	Imperceptible	Barely perceptible	Flat areola, no bud	Stippled areola: 1- to 2-mm bud	Raised areola; 3- to 4-mm bud	Full areola; 5- to 10-mm bud	–	
Eye and ear	Lids fused, loosely: -1; tightly: -2	Lids open; pinna flat, stays folded	Slightly curved pinna; soft slow recoil	Well-curved pinna; soft but ready recoil	Formed and firm; instant recoil	Thick cartilage; ear stiff	–	
Genitalia (male)	Scrotum flat, smooth	Scrotum empty; faint rugae	Testes in upper canal; rare rugae	Testes descending; few rugae	Testes down; good rugae	Testes pendulous; deep rugae	–	
Genitalia (female)	Clitoris prominent; labia flat	Prominent clitoris; small labia minora	Prominent clitoris; enlarging minora	Majora and minora equally prominent	Majora large; minora small	Majora cover clitoris and minora	–	

Total physical maturity score

MATURITY RATING

Physical Maturity Score	-10	-5	0	5	10	15	20	25	30	35	40	45	50
Gestational Age (weeks)	20	22	24	26	28	30	32	34	36	38	40	42	44

SCORE

Neuromuscular _____

Physical _____

Total _____

GESTATIONAL AGE (weeks)

By dates _____

By ultrasound _____

By score _____

Reproduced from Ballard, J. L., "New Ballard Score Expanded to Include Extremely Premature Infants,"
Journal of Pediatrics 119:417-23, 1991, with permission of Mosby-Year Book, Inc.

♦ **III. Neonatal physical examination**

A. Head
   1. The neonate's head is approximately one-fourth of body size
   2. *Molding* refers to asymmetry of the skull from overriding of cranial sutures during labor and delivery
   3. *Cephalhematoma* is the collection of blood between a skull bone and the periosteum that does not cross suture lines
   4. *Caput succedaneum* is localized swelling over the presenting part that can cross suture lines

B. Fontanels
   1. The diamond-shaped anterior fontanel is located at the juncture of the frontal and parietal bones
      a. It measures 1⅛″ to 1⅝″ (3 to 4 cm) long and ¾″ to 1⅛″ (2 to 3 cm) wide
      b. It closes in approximately 18 months
   2. The triangular-shaped posterior fontanel is located at the juncture of the occipital and parietal bones
      a. It measures approximately 2 cm across
      b. It closes in approximately 8 to 12 weeks
   3. The fontanels should feel soft to the touch

      a. A depressed fontanel indicates dehydration
      b. Bulging fontanel requires immediate attention because it may indicate increased intracranial pressure

C. Eyes
   1. The neonate's eyes are usually blue or gray because of scleral thinness
   2. Permanent eye color is established in 3 to 12 months
   3. Lacrimal glands are immature at birth, resulting in tearless crying for up to 2 months
   4. The neonate may demonstrate transient STRABISMUS
   5. DOLL'S EYE PHENOMENON may persist for about 10 days
   6. Subconjunctival hemorrhages may appear from vascular tension changes during birth

D. Nose
   1. Infants are obligatory nose-breathers for the first few months of life
   2. Nasal passages must be kept clear to ensure adequate respirations
   3. Neonates instinctively sneeze to remove obstruction

E. Mouth
   1. EPSTEIN'S PEARLS may be found on the gums or hard palate
   2. The neonate usually has scant saliva and pink lips
   3. Precocious teeth may appear

F. Ears
1. The neonate's ears are characterized by incurving of the pinna and cartilage deposition
2. The top of the ear should be above or parallel to an imaginary line from the inner to outer canthus of the eye
3. Low-set ears are associated with several syndromes, including chromosomal abnormalities

G. Neck
1. The neonate's neck is typically short and weak
2. It has deep skin folds

H. Chest
1. Cylindrical thorax and flexible ribs are characteristic at birth
2. Breast engorgement may occur from maternal hormones
3. Extra nipples (supernumerary) may be located below and medially to the true nipples

I. Abdomen
1. The abdomen is usually cylindrical, with some protrusion
2. A scaphoid appearance indicates diaphragmatic hernia

J. Umbilical cord
1. The cord is white and gelatinous, with two arteries and one vein
2. It begins to dry within 1 to 2 hours after delivery

K. Genitals
1. In males, rugae appear on the scrotum; testes are descended into the scrotum; and the urinary meatus is located at the penile tip (normal), on the dorsal surface (epispadias), or on the ventral surface (hypospadias)
2. In females, labia majora cover the labia minora and clitoris, vaginal discharge from maternal hormones appears, and the hymenal tag is present

L. Extremities
1. All neonates are bowlegged and have flat feet
2. The neonate may have abnormal extremities
   a. Polydactyl: more than five digits on an extremity
   b. Syndactyl: fusing together of two or more digits

M. Back
1. The spine should be straight and flat
2. NEVUS PILOSUS at the base of the spine is commonly associated with spina bifida

N. Anus: normally patent without any fissure

O. Skin

1. The neonate may exhibit acrocyanosis (cyanosis of the hands and feet resulting from adjustments to extrauterine circulation)
2. Milia are clogged sebaceous glands, usually on the nose or chin
3. Lanugo is fine, downy hair found after 20 weeks of gestation on the entire body except the palms and soles
4. Vernix caseosa is a white cheesy protective coating composed of desquamated epithelial cells and sebum
5. Erythema neonatorum toxicum is a transient, maculopapular rash
6. Telangiectasia (flat, reddened vascular areas) may appear on the neck, upper eyelid, or upper lip
7. Port-wine stain (nevus flammeus), a capillary angioma located below the dermis and commonly found on the face, is a flat, sharply demarcated purple-red birthmark
8. Strawberry mark (nevus vasculosus), a capillary angioma located in the dermal and subdermal skin layers, is a rough, raised, sharply demarcated birthmark

P. Reflexes

1. Sucking: sucking motion begins when a nipple is placed in the neonate's mouth
2. Moro's reflex: when the neonate is lifted above the crib and then suddenly lowered, the arms and legs symmetrically extend, then abduct; the fingers spread, forming a "C"
3. Rooting: stroking the cheek makes the neonate turn the head in the direction of the stroke
4. Tonic neck (fencing position): when the neonate is supine and the head is turned to one side, extremities on the same side straighten while those on the opposite side flex
5. Babinski's reflex: stroking the sole on the side of the small toe makes the toes fan upward
6. Grasping: placing a finger in each hand makes the neonate grasp the fingers tightly enough to be pulled to a sitting position
7. Stepping: holding the neonate upright with the feet touching a flat surface elicits dancing or stepping movements
8. Startle: a loud noise, such as a hand clap, elicits arm abduction and elbow flexion; the hands stay clenched
9. Trunk incurvature: when a finger is run down the neonate's back, laterally to the spine, the trunk flexes and the pelvis swings toward the stimulated side

♦ **IV. Behavioral assessment**

A. Sensory behaviors: Tactile
1. Sensations of pressure, pain, and touch are present at birth or soon after
2. Lips are hypersensitive
3. Skin on thighs, forearms, and trunk is hyposensitive
4. The neonate is especially sensitive to being cuddled and touched

B. Sensory behaviors: Olfactory
1. The neonate can differentiate pleasant from unpleasant odors after mucus and amniotic fluid have been cleared from nasal passages
2. The neonate can distinguish the mother's wet breast pad from those of other mothers at age 1 week

C. Sensory behaviors: Vision
1. The neonate can see approximately 7″ to 8″ (17.5 to 20 cm) at birth
2. Eyes have immature muscle control and coordination
3. Eyes are sensitive to light
4. The neonate can track the parent's eyes
5. The neonate prefers complex patterns in black and white

D. Sensory behaviors: Auditory: the neonate can detect sounds at birth

E. Sensory behaviors: Taste
1. Taste buds develop before birth
2. The neonate prefers sweet tastes to bitter or sour ones

F. Behavioral assessment
1. Period of reactivity
   a. Lasts about 30 minutes after birth
   b. The neonate is awake and active and may demonstrate sucking reflex
   c. Respiratory rate and heart rate increase
   d. It is an ideal time to initiate parental-infant bonding and breast-feeding
2. Sleep phase
   a. Lasts from several minutes to 2 to 4 hours
   b. Pulse rate and respiratory rate return to baseline
3. Second period of reactivity
   a. Lasts 4 to 6 hours
   b. Pulse rate and respiratory rate increase again

♦ **V. Nutrition**

A. General information
1. Neonates lose approximately 10% of birthweight in the first few days of extrauterine life but usually regain it within 10 days

2. Infants typically gain 1 oz (28 g) per day in the first 6 months and ½ oz (14 g) per day in the second 6 months

3. Most infants double their birthweight by age 6 months and triple it by age 1 year

4. The American Academy of Pediatrics recommends that formula-fed infants be given an iron supplement for the first year

B. Daily nutritional requirements

1. Calories: 95 to 145 kcal/kg
2. Protein: 2.2 g/kg in the first 6 months; 2 g/kg in the second 6 months
3. Fluid: 130 to 200 ml/kg

C. Breast-feeding

1. Advantages
   a. Is economical
   b. Is readily available
   c. Promotes development of facial muscles, jaw, and teeth
   d. Aids in uterine involution
   e. Promotes transfer of maternal antibodies
   f. Enhances maternal-infant bonding
   g. Is nutritionally superior to all other options
   h. Reduces incidence of allergies
   i. Reduces incidence of maternal breast cancer

2. Disadvantages
   a. Prevents others from feeding the infant unless milk is expressed or pumped
   b. Limits the paternal role in infant feeding
   c. Compels the mother to monitor her diet carefully
   d. May be difficult for a working mother to maintain

D. Bottle-feeding

1. Advantages
   a. Permits the father and other family members to feed the infant
   b. Poses fewer restrictions on the mother than breast-feeding
   c. Allows more accurate measuring of intake
   d. Enables the mother to take medications without risk to the infant
   e. Requires fewer feedings than breast-feeding
   f. Enables the mother to feed the infant in public without embarrassment

2. Disadvantages
   a. Costs more than breast-feeding
   b. Requires greater preparation time and effort
   c. Requires cleanliness of hands, water, and equipment
   d. Requires adequate refrigeration and storage
   e. Does not promote transfer of maternal antibodies
   f. Does not benefit the mother physiologically

◆ VI. General infant care

A. Provide appropriate care after circumcision

1. Observe and record the first void after circumcision
2. Apply a thin layer of petroleum gauze to the site to control bleeding and prevent the diaper from adhering to the penis
3. Wash the penis gently with water, and apply fresh petroleum gauze to the glans with each diaper change
4. Apply gentle pressure with a sterile 4″ × 4″ gauze pad if bleeding occurs; notify the doctor if bleeding continues

B. Use proper cleaning and bathing techniques

1. Give the first bath when vital signs have stabilized
2. Give the neonate a sponge bath until the umbilical cord falls off
3. Use a mild, hexachlorophene-free soap
4. Do not use soap on the face
5. Wash, rinse, and dry each portion of the body separately to minimize heat loss
6. Bathe before feedings instead of afterwards to prevent vomiting

C. Position and hold the infant properly

1. Position the infant comfortably (commonly on the side, with a rolled blanket supporting the back)
2. Position the infant on the right side after feeding to enhance gastric emptying
3. Teach the mother the football hold, which provides adequate support for the infant while freeing a hand (For more teaching tips, see *Parental care of the normal neonate,* page 112)

D. Change the infant's diaper before and immediately after feeding

1. Place the diaper below the umbilical cord to prevent contamination
2. Gently clean an uncircumcised penis; do not attempt to retract the foreskin
3. Wipe the vulva of a female infant from front to back to avoid rectal contamination of the urethra or vagina

E. Maintain normal body temperature (97.7° to 98.6° F [36.5° to 37° C])

1. Take an axillary temperature every shift after temperature stabilizes
2. Apply a cap to the neonate's head to prevent heat loss
3. Single- or double-wrap the infant snugly
4. Avoid exposing the infant to drafts, wetness, and direct or indirect contact with cold surfaces

TEACHING TIPS
Parental care of the normal neonate

Be sure to include the following topics in your teaching plan for the parents of a normal neonate:
- Normal newborn characteristics and physical behaviors
- Umbilical stump care
- Bathing techniques
- Feeding and burping
- Proper positioning and holding
- Circumcision care, if appropriate
- Diapering
- Methods to check for jaundice at home if discharged early

F. Check the neonate's pulse and respiratory rates frequently until they stabilize; then take an apical pulse and monitor respirations once every shift

G. Suction the nose and mouth as needed; have a bulb syringe available to remove excessive mucus or milk from air passages promptly

Points to remember

◆ The neonate must undergo major multi-system adjustments during the transition from intrauterine to extrauterine existence.

◆ To perform a comprehensive assessment of the neonate, the nurse must assess both physical and behavioral characteristics.

◆ The ideal time to initiate parent-neonate bonding is within the first 30 minutes after birth.

◆ All of the neonate's senses are functional at birth.

Study questions

To evaluate your understanding of this chapter, answer the following questions in the space provided; then compare your responses with the correct answers in Appendix B, page 174.

1. When is the Apgar score performed? _____

_____

_____

2. Which method should the nurse use when taking the neonate's temperature for the first time? Why? _____

_____

_____

3. Which major changes occur in the cardiovascular system as the neonate adapts to extrauterine existence? _____

_____

_____

4. When would the nurse expect the anterior and posterior fontanels to close?

_____

_____

5. How would the nurse elicit Moro's reflex? _____

_____

_____

6. Which neonate behaviors and physiologic events characterize the period of reactivity? _____

_____

_____

7. What are the daily nutritional requirements of an infant?_____

_____

_____

CRITICAL THINKING AND APPLICATION EXERCISES

1. Using the Ballard Gestational Age Assessment Tool, perform a gestational age assessment on a neonate.

2. Prepare an instruction sheet for parents taking their neonate home.

3. Follow a neonate from delivery through discharge. Develop a patient-specific plan of care, including any needs for parental education and neonatal follow-up.

CHAPTER

9

The High-Risk Neonate

LEARNING OBJECTIVES

After studying this chapter, you should be able to:

♦ State the signs of respiratory distress syndrome in the newborn.

♦ Identify potential complications in high-risk neonates.

♦ Identify clinical manifestations of drug addiction in the newborn.

♦ Discuss the effect of maternal infectious diseases upon the fetus or neonate.

♦ Describe the physical characteristics of a premature, post-mature, small-for-gestational age, and large-for-gestational age infant.

CHAPTER OVERVIEW

Some neonates experience conditions that complicate the neonatal period or place the neonate at high risk of present and future problems. Knowledge of the pathophysiology and contributing factors allows for early identification and prompt management of these conditions which is vital to prevent or minimize long-term effects.

◆ I. Respiratory distress syndrome

A. General information
1. Also called hyaline membrane disease
2. A complex disorder manifested by signs of respiratory distress

B. Pathophysiology
1. Inability to synthesize sufficient surfactant
2. Unable to maintain alveolar stability

C. Clinical manifestations
1. Tachypnea
2. Nasal flaring
3. Grunting
4. Retractions
5. Bilateral diffuse reticulogranular density on X-ray

D. Assessment
1. Silverman-Anderson index to evaluate respiratory status (see *Silverman-Anderson index,* page 116)
2. Five areas graded on a scale of 0 to 2

E. Management
1. Ventilatory therapy
2. Maintenance of acid-base balance
3. Temperature regulation
4. Adequate nutrition
5. Transcutaneous oxygen monitoring
6. Administration of surfactant
7. Protection from infection

◆ II. Transient tachypnea of the newborn (TTN)

A. General information
1. Also known as Type II respiratory distress syndrome
2. A progressive respiratory distress

B. Pathophysiology
1. Aspiration of amniotic or tracheal fluid compounded either by delayed clearing of the airway or by excess fluid entering the lungs
2. Spontaneously fades as lung fluid is absorbed, usually by 72 hours of life, as respiratory activity becomes effective

C. Clinical manifestations
1. Expiratory grunting
2. Nasal flaring
3. Slight cyanosis
4. Tachypnea

Silverman-Anderson index

Used to evaluate the neonate's respiratory status, the Silverman-Anderson index assesses five areas: upper chest, lower chest, xiphoid retractions, nares dilation, and expiratory grunt. Each area is graded 0 (no respiratory difficulty), 1 (moderate difficulty), or 2 (maximum difficulty), with a total score ranging from 0 (no respiratory difficulty) to 10 (maximal respiratory difficulty).

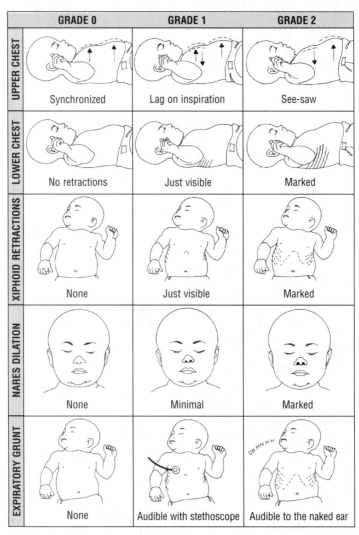

	GRADE 0	GRADE 1	GRADE 2
UPPER CHEST	Synchronized	Lag on inspiration	See-saw
LOWER CHEST	No retractions	Just visible	Marked
XIPHOID RETRACTIONS	None	Just visible	Marked
NARES DILATION	None	Minimal	Marked
EXPIRATORY GRUNT	None	Audible with stethoscope	Audible to the naked ear

From Silverman, W.A., and Anderson, D.H. *Pediatrics* 17(1), 1956. Used with permission.

D. Management
1. Oxygen administration
2. Ventilatory assistance (rarely needed)
3. Maintenance of acid-base balance
4. Thermoregulation
5. Adequate nutrition
6. Transcutaneous oxygen monitoring
7. Protection from infection

◆ III. Meconium aspiration syndrome

A. General information
1. Aspiration of meconium into the lungs
2. Possibly occurring before or at delivery

B. Pathophysiology
1. Asphyxia in utero leads to increased fetal peristalsis, relaxation of the anal sphincter, passage of meconium into the amniotic fluid, and reflex gasping of amniotic fluid into the lungs
2. Meconium creates a ball-valve effect, trapping air in the alveolus and preventing adequate gas exchange
3. Chemical pneumonitis results, causing the alveolar walls and interstitial tissues to thicken, again preventing adequate gas exchange
4. Cardiac efficiency can be compromised from pulmonary hypertension

C. Clinical manifestations
1. Fetal hypoxia as indicated by altered fetal activity and heart rate
2. Meconium staining of amniotic fluid noted on rupture of membranes
3. Signs of distress at delivery, such as Apgar scores below 6, pallor, cyanosis, and respiratory distress

D. Management
1. Immediate endotracheal suctioning of the neonate at delivery
2. Respiratory assistance via mechanical ventilation
3. Maintenance of a neutral thermal environment
4. Postural drainage
5. Chest physiotherapy
6. Administration of antibiotics

◆ IV. Sepsis

A. General information
1. Pathogenic microorganisms or their toxins in the blood or tissues
2. Can occur before, during, or after delivery

3. Most common causative agents are the gram-negative *Escherichia coli, Aerobacter, Proteus,* and *Klebsiella* and the gram-positive beta-hemolytic streptococci

B. Clinical manifestations
1. Subtle, nonspecific behavioral changes, such as lethargy or hypotonia
2. Temperature instability
3. Feeding pattern changes, such as poor sucking or decreased intake
4. Apnea
5. Hyperbilirubinemia
6. Abdominal distention

C. General management
1. Collection of specimens to identify causative organisms
2. Lumbar puncture
3. Urine, skin, blood, and nasopharyngeal cultures
4. Gastric aspiration

D. Nursing management
1. Administration of broad-spectrum antibiotics before culture results are received; specific antibiotic therapy after results are received
2. Physiologic supportive care, including maintenance of a neutral thermal environment
3. Respiratory support
4. Evaluation of signs and symptoms of sepsis
5. Monitoring of fluid and electrolyte balance
6. Evaluation of metabolic disturbances
7. Provision for cardiovascular support

♦ V. Hyperbilirubinemia (pathologic jaundice)

A. General information
1. Condition characterized by a bilirubin level that exceeds 6 mg/dl within the first 24 hours after delivery and remains elevated beyond 7 days in a full-term neonate and 10 days in a premature neonate
2. A bilirubin level that rises by more than 5 mg/day
3. A level that is greater than 12 mg/dl in premature or term neonates
4. Conjugated (direct) bilirubin level that exceeds 1.5 to 2 mg/dl

B. Pathophysiology
1. Unconjugated bilirubin can infiltrate the nuclei of the cerebral cortex and thalamus, leading to kernicterus (an encephalopathy)
2. Kernicterus may occur with serum bilirubin levels at or above 20 mg/dl (full-term) and at lower levels (approximately 14 mg/dl) in premature neonates

3. Signs of kernicterus: lethargy, decreased reflexes, seizures, opistho-
tonos, and high-pitched cry
4. Possible causes may include: hemolytic disease of the neonate, sepsis, impaired hepatic functioning, polycythemia, enclosed hemorrhage, hypothermia, hypoglycemia, and asphyxia neonatorum

C. Clinical manifestations
1. Jaundice
2. Elevated bilirubin levels
3. Hepatosplenomegaly

D. Management
1. Treatment for anemia caused by hemolytic disease

**CLINICAL
ALERT**

2. Increased serum albumin levels
3. Removal of maternal antibodies and sensitized red blood cells via exchange transfusion and phototherapy

◆ VI. Isoimmune hemolytic disease of the neonate

A. General information
1. Formerly called erythroblastosis fetalis
2. Involves a breakdown of red blood cells

B. Pathophysiology
1. Transplacental passage of maternal antibodies that causes red blood
cell breakdown
2. Most often caused by ABO incompatibility; may be caused by Rh
incompatibility
a. ABO incompatibility can occur when fetal blood type differs
from maternal blood type
(1) The most common incompatibility occurs when a type O
mother carries a type A or type B fetus; type O blood contains anti-A and anti-B antibodies that travel transplacentally to the fetus, causing jaundice and hepatosplenomegaly
(2) ABO incompatibility can occur with the first pregnancy and
is usually milder and of shorter duration than Rh incompatibility
b. Rh incompatibility occurs when an Rh-negative mother carries
an Rh-positive fetus
(1) Leakage of fetal Rh antigens commonly occurs during delivery, at the time of placental separation
(2) Maternal antibodies are produced in response; in a subsequent pregnancy with an Rh-positive fetus, maternal antibodies enter the fetal circulation transplacentally, causing
erythroblastosis

C. Clinical manifestations
   1. Hemolytic anemia
   2. Hyperbilirubinemia
   3. Jaundice
   4. Hepatosplenomegaly

D. Management
   1. Drug therapy
   2. Family support
   3. Phototherapy
   4. Exchange transfusion
   5. Monitoring of bilirubin levels

E. Prevention
   1. Prevention involves administration of Rh immune globulin (RhoGAM) within 72 hours of delivery
   2. RhoGAM prevents antibody formation

CLINICAL ALERT
   3. RhoGAM is ineffective when the woman is already sensitized
   4. RhoGAM should be administered to an Rh-negative, D_u-negative woman who has had an abortion or whose newborn is Rh positive or D_u positive

CLINICAL ALERT
   5. Rh sensitization can occur during pregnancy if the cellular layer separating maternal and fetal circulation is disrupted
   6. RhoGAM can be administered at 28 weeks of gestation to decrease the incidence of maternal isoimmunizations

◆ **VII. Fetal alcohol syndrome (FAS)**

A. General information

CLINICAL ALERT
   1. This disorder is commonly found in newborns of women who ingested varying amounts of alcohol during pregnancy
   2. Alcohol is a teratogenic substance of particular danger during critical periods of organogenesis
   3. Alcohol interferes with the passage of amino acids across the placental barrier

B. Clinical manifestations
   1. Prenatal and postnatal growth retardation
   2. Facial anomalies (microcephaly, microophthalmia, maxillary hypoplasia, short palpebral fissures)
   3. Central nervous system dysfunction (decreased I.Q., developmental delays, neurologic abnormalities)

C. Risk factors

CLINICAL ALERT
   1. The risk of teratogenic effects increases proportionally with increased daily alcohol intake
   2. No safe level of alcohol intake during pregnancy has been established

3. FAS has been detected in neonates of moderate drinkers (1 to 2 oz of alcohol daily)

   D. Management

     1. Prevention through public education

     2. Careful prenatal history and education

     3. Identification of women at risk, with referral to alcohol treatment centers if necessary

♦ VIII. Drug addiction

   A. Clinical manifestations

     1. High-pitched cry

     2. Jitteriness

     3. Tremors

     4. Irritability

     5. Poor feeding habits

     6. Hyperactive Moro's reflex

     7. Increased tendon reflexes

     8. Frequent sneezing and yawning

     9. Poor sleeping pattern

    10. Diarrhea

    11. Vigorous sucking on hands

   B. Withdrawal

     1. Manifestations of withdrawal depend on the length of maternal addiction, the drug ingested, and the time of last ingestion before delivery

     2. Withdrawal usually occurs within 24 hours of delivery

   C. Management

     1. Tight swaddling for comfort

     2. A quiet, dark environment to decrease environmental stimuli

     3. A pacifier to meet sucking needs (heroin withdrawal)

     4. Gavage feeding for poor sucking reflex (methadone withdrawal)

     5. Maintenance of fluid and electrolyte balance

     6. Avoidance of breast-feeding

     7. Assessment for jaundice (methadone withdrawal)

     8. Medication to treat withdrawal signs (paregoric and phenobarbital [Barbita])

     9. Promotion of maternal-infant bonding

    10. Evaluation for referral to child protective services, if warranted

   D. Contraindications: methadone should not be given to newborns because of its addictive nature

◆ IX. Sexually transmitted diseases

A. Syphilis
1. Assessment
   a. Congenital syphilis is diagnosed with serologic tests at 3 to 6 months
   b. The development of antibodies is necessary to make a diagnosis
2. Clinical manifestations
   a. Vesicular lesions on the soles and palms
   b. Irritability
   c. Small for gestational age
   d. Failure to thrive
   e. Rhinitis
   f. Red rash around mouth and anus
   g. Copper rash on face, soles, and palms
3. Management
   a. Penicillin therapy
   b. Isolation technique initially, followed by general care
   c. Covering of hands to minimize skin trauma from scratching

B. Gonorrhea
1. Etiology: exposure to lesion during vaginal delivery
2. Clinical manifestation: ophthalmia neonatorum
3. Management
   a. Penicillin therapy
   b. Prophylactic medication administration, such as erythromycin, to the eyes after delivery
   c. Isolation measures
   d. Culture specimens of eye discharge, if present

◆ X. Hydrocephaly

A. General information
1. Abnormal increase in the amount of cerebrospinal fluid (CSF) in the ventricles of the brain
2. Can lead to cerebral ventricle enlargement

B. Pathophysiology
1. Alteration in production (increased), flow (obstructed), or reabsorption of CSF
2. Resultant increase in intracranial pressure causing brain displacement, motor and mental damage

C. Clinical manifestations
1. Head enlargement
2. Forehead prominence
3. "Sunset eyes"

4. Irritability
5. Weakness
6. Seizures

D. Management
1. Skin care to prevent breakdown and infection
2. Careful head support during handling
3. Emotional support and education for the parents
4. Assessment of neurologic status and progression of symptoms
5. Shunt insertion to eliminate excess CSF
6. Management of shunt and prevention of infection at the surgical site

◆ XI. Phenylketonuria (PKU)

A. General information
1. Inborn metabolic error
2. Deficiency of phenylalanine hydroxylase, a liver enzyme essential for the conversion of phenylalanine to tyrosine

B. Pathophysiology
1. Accumulation of phenylalanine and its abnormal metabolites in the brain
2. Possibly leading to mental retardation

C. Clinical manifestations
1. Failure to thrive
2. Vomiting
3. Rashes
4. Decreased pigmentation

CLINICAL ALERT

D. Management
1. The Guthrie test, using a heel stick, is required by most states and should be performed at least 24 hours after initiation of feedings
2. Infants are placed on low-phenylalanine formula (Lofenalac) and on a continued special diet that limits phenylalanine intake
3. Central nervous system damage can be minimized if treatment is initiated before age 3 months

◆ XII. TORCH syndrome

A. General information
1. Group of maternal infectious diseases (*TO*xoplasmosis, *R*ubella, *C*ytomegalovirus, *H*erpesvirus Type II)
2. Can lead to serious complications in the embryo, fetus, and neonate

B. Toxoplasmosis
1. The disease is transmitted to the fetus primarily via the mother's contact with contaminated cat box filler

2. A therapeutic abortion is recommended if the diagnosis is made before the 20th week of gestation
3. Effects include increased frequency of stillbirths, neonatal deaths, severe congenital anomalies, retinochoroiditis, seizures, and coma

C. Rubella
1. This chronic viral infection lasts from the first trimester to months after delivery
2. The greatest risk occurs within the first trimester
3. Effects include congenital heart disease, intrauterine growth retardation, cataracts, mental retardation, and hearing impairment
4. Management includes therapeutic abortion if the disease occurs during the first trimester, and emotional support for parents
5. Women of childbearing age should be tested for immunity and vaccinated if necessary

D. Cytomegalovirus (CMV)
1. CMV is a member of the herpesvirus group that can be transmitted from an asymptomatic mother transplacentally to the fetus or via the cervix to the neonate at delivery
2. It is the most frequent cause of viral infections in the fetus
3. CMV is a common cause of mental retardation
4. Principal sites of damage are the brain, liver, and blood
5. Other effects include auditory difficulties and a birth weight that is small for gestational age
6. Antiviral drugs cannot prevent CMV or treat the neonate

E. Herpesvirus Type II
1. The fetus can be exposed to the herpesvirus through indirect contact with infected genitals or via direct contact with those tissues during delivery
2. Affected neonates may be asymptomatic for 2 to 12 days but then may develop jaundice, seizures, increased temperature, and characteristic vesicular lesions
3. A cesarean delivery can protect the fetus from infection

◆ XIII. Cleft lip and palate

A. General information
1. Cleft lip refers to an incomplete fusion of upper lip
2. Cleft palate is an opening in the palate; may involve the hard or soft palate or both

B. Pathophysiology
1. Cleft lip occurs when the maxillary and median nose processes fail to close during embryonic development

2. Cleft palate results when the sides of the palate do not fuse during embryonic development

C. Clinical Manifestations
   1. Both conditions may be either unilateral or bilateral
   2. Cleft lip is readily obvious at birth
      a. A small notch in the upper lip to a total separation of lip and facial structure up into the floor of the nose
      b. Flattened nose
      c. Possible absent teeth and gingiva
   3. Entire palate must be carefully inspected; opening on hard or soft palate

D. Management
   1. Surgical correction of cleft lip several weeks after birth and cleft palate at 12 to 18 months
   2. Emotional support to parents
   3. Evaluation for special feeding devices, such as preemie or cleft palate nipple
   4. Feeding in high Fowler's position
   5. Burping every ½ to 1 oz
   6. Follow-up feeding with water to clear nasal passages
   7. Parent instruction regarding increased incidence of speech defects and upper respiratory infections as the infant grows

♦ XIV. Retinopathy of prematurity (ROP)

A. General information
   1. Alteration in vision leading to partial or total blindness
   2. Resulting from prolonged exposure to high concentrations of oxygen

B. Pathophysiology
   1. High oxygen concentrations leads to vasoconstriction of immature retinal blood vessels
   2. Subsequent rupture of vessels with partial or complete retinal detachment

C. Clinical manifestations: retinal changes upon ophthalmologic examination

D. Management
   1. Monitoring oxygen concentrations
   2. Monitoring arterial blood gases
   3. Monitoring of oxygenation with a pulse oximeter
   4. Ophthalmologic examinations at regular intervals during and following hospitalization

5. Administration of Vitamin E (reduces incidence of ROP by modifying tissues' response to effects of oxygen)

♦ XV. Tracheoesophageal fistula

A. General information

1. Congenital anomaly resulting from some teratogen not allowing esophagus and trachea to separate normally
2. Abnormal connection between the trachea and esophagus

B. Pathophysiology

1. Abnormal development of the trachea and esophagus during the embryonic period
2. Most frequently, esophagus ends in blind pouch with trachea communicating by a fistula with lower esophagus and stomach

C. Clinical manifestations

1. Signs of respiratory distress
2. Excessive mucous secretions
3. Difficulty passing a nasogastric tube
4. Difficulty feeding; that is, choking or aspiration

D. Management

1. Maintenance of patent airway
2. Surgical correction
3. Position in high-Fowler's to prevent aspirations of gastric contents
4. Laryngoscope and endotracheal tube at bedside in case of extreme edema causing obstruction
5. Frequent shallow suctioning
6. Pacifier to meet sucking needs
7. Possible gastrostomy tube feedings postoperatively

CLINICAL ALERT

♦ XVI. Congenital hip dysplasia

A. General information

1. Improper formation and function of the hip socket
2. Tendency of the head of the femur to ride out of or dislocate from the acetabulum

B. Pathophysiology

1. Exact cause unknown
2. The acetabulum too shallow, thus allowing the head of the femur to become dislocated upward and backward

C. Clinical manifestations

1. Positive Ortolani's sign
2. Shortened femur on affected side
3. Asymmetrical gluteal folds

D. Interventions
　　1. Positioning and maintaining head of femur in acetabulum by triple diapers, Frejka pillow splint, or Pavlik harness
　　2. Hip spica cast and braces if other means ineffective
　　3. Parent education about use of device for maintaining position

◆ **XVII. Apnea of the newborn**

A. General information
　　1. Cessation of breathing for greater than 15 to 20 seconds
　　2. Commonly seen in preterm infants and infants with secondary stress, such as those with infection, hyperbilirubinemia, hypoglycemia, or hypothermia

B. Pathophysiology
　　1. Immaturity of respiratory centers in the brain
　　2. Insufficient amounts of surfactant
　　3. Acidosis
　　4. Anemia
　　5. Hypoglycemia or hyperglycemia
　　6. Hypothermia or hyperthermia
　　7. Upper airway obstruction
　　8. Hypocalcemia
　　9. Sepsis

C. Clinical manifestations
　　1. Cessation of breathing greater than 15 to 20 seconds
　　2. Bradycardia
　　3. Early cyanosis

D. Interventions
　　1. Respiratory support
　　2. Tactile stimulation
　　3. Correction of underlying cause; i.e., hypoglycemia
　　4. Gentle handling
　　5. Evaluation of blood gas levels
　　6. Suctioning
　　7. Home apnea monitoring (For teaching tips, see *Home apnea monitoring,* page 128)

◆ **XVIII. Prematurity**

A. General information
　　1. Delivery before the end of the 37th week of gestation
　　2. Problems associated with prematurity: immaturity of all systems; extent depends on gestational age and level of development at delivery

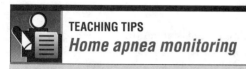

TEACHING TIPS
Home apnea monitoring

Be sure to include the following topics in your teaching plan for the parents of a neonate receiving home apnea monitoring:
- Rationale for use
- Signs and symptoms of apnea
- Equipment and procedure for use
- Frequency and duration of use
- Signs and symptoms to notify doctor
- Measures to stimulate respirations
- Cardiopulmonary resuscitation technique
- Follow-up care

      3. Premature neonates between 28 and 37 weeks have the best chance of survival

B. Management
    1. Respiratory assessment and assistance
    2. Maintenance of fluid and electrolyte balance
    3. Prevention of infection
    4. Assessment of neurologic status
    5. Maintenance of body temperature and neutral thermal environment
    6. Renal function monitoring
    7. Emotional support to parents
    8. Assessment of glucose and bilirubin levels

♦ XIX. Small for gestational age (SGA)

A. General information
    1. Birth weight at or below the 10th percentile on intrauterine growth chart
    2. Also referred to as small-for-dates and intrauterine growth retardation

B. Maternal causes
    1. Poor nutrition
    2. Advanced diabetes
    3. Pregnancy-induced hypertension
    4. Smoking
    5. Age over 35
    6. Drug use

C. Placental causes: partial placental separation and malfunction

D. Fetal causes
   1. Intrauterine infection
   2. Chromosomal abnormalities and malformations

E. Problems associated with SGA
   1. Perinatal asphyxia
   2. Hypoglycemia
   3. Hypocalcemia
   4. Aspiration syndromes
   5. Increased heat loss
   6. Feeding difficulties
   7. Polycythemia

F. Clinical manifestations
   1. Wide-eyed look
   2. Sunken abdomen
   3. Loose, dry skin
   4. Decreased chest and abdomen circumferences
   5. Decreased subcutaneous fat
   6. Thin, dry umbilical cord
   7. Sparse scalp hair

G. Management: see Section XVIII, B

◆ XX. Large for gestational age (LGA)

A. General information
   1. Birthweight at or above the 90th percentile on the intrauterine growth chart
   2. Subjected to an overproduction of growth hormone in utero

B. Etiology
   1. Mother with poorly controlled diabetes
   2. Multiparity
   3. Infant with transposition of the great vessels (unknown cause)
   4. Genetic predisposition

C. Problems associated with LGA
   1. Increased incidence of cesarean deliveries, birth trauma, and injury
   2. Hypoglycemia
   3. Polycythemia

D. Management: see Section XVIII, B

◆ XXI. Postmaturity

A. General information
   1. Delivery after 42 weeks of gestation

2. Placenta with growth potential for only 40 to 42 weeks; after that time, calcium deposits collect, making placenta unable to function resulting in fetus possibly suffering from lack of oxygen, fluids, and nutrients

B. Etiology
1. Not well understood
2. Associated with primigravidas, anencephalic fetus, history of post-maturity, and delayed ovulation and fertilization

C. Problems associated with postmaturity
1. Meconium aspiration
2. Placental insufficiency
3. Hypoxia
4. Hypoglycemia
5. Polycythemia
6. Seizures
7. Cold stress

**CLINICAL
ALERT**

D. Clinical manifestations
1. Alert, wide-eyed look
2. Absence of vernix caseosa
3. Long fingernails
4. Profuse scalp hair
5. Long, thin body
6. Decreased or absent subcutaneous fat
7. Loose, dry skin
8. Meconium

E. Management: see Section XVIII, B

◆ XXII. Human immunodeficiency virus (HIV) infection

A. General information
1. Infectious disease caused by HIV compromising the immune system
2. Acquired by fetus transplacentally through contact with maternal blood or secretions and breast milk
3. Diagnosis determined by lab testing, evidence of immunosuppression, wasting syndrome, encephalopathy, and opportunistic diseases

**CLINICAL
ALERT**

4. Note: False positive test for HIV antibodies may result from trans-placental transfer of maternal HIV antibodies to the fetus; final diagnosis may take up to 6 months

B. Clinical manifestations
1. Recurrent infections
2. SGA status
3. Oral candidiasis (thrush)
4. Lymphoid interstitial pneumonia

     5. Facial dysmorphism (boxy forehead; increased inner and outer canthal distance; flat, broad nasal bridge; spreading lips; and prominent triangular philtrum)

     6. Hepatosplenomegaly

     7. Failure to thrive

C. Management

     1. See Section XVIII, B

     2. Drug therapy with AZT 2 mg/kg PO every 6 hours for 6 weeks

For more information, see Chapter 11, Complications and High-Risk Conditions of the Postpartum Period.

◆ XXIII. Seizures

A. General information

     1. Typically a symptom of an underlying disorder

     2. May be caused by perinatal injury, effects of anoxia, or metabolic disease; susceptible neonates include those who have experienced severe asphyxia, intracranial hemorrhage, or acute drug withdrawal

B. Clinical manifestations

     1. Subtle signs include nystagmus, repeated blinking, sucking motions, and tongue thrusting

     2. Obvious signs include rhythmic movements of extremities and rigid posture

**CLINICAL
ALERT**

     3. Suspected seizure activity must be differentiated from jitteriness; holding the affected extremity will stop jitteriness but not true seizures

C. Management

     1. Correction of underlying cause

     2. Maintenance of patent airway

     3. See also Section XVIII, B

POINTS TO REMEMBER

◆ Signs of respiratory distress must be reported immediately; they include tachypnea, respiratory grunting, nasal flaring, retractions, and cyanosis.

◆ Meconium aspiration may occur before or at delivery.

◆ Kernicterus may occur with bilirubin levels above 20 mg/dl in full-term neonates.

◆ Isoimmune hemolytic disease most often is caused by ABO incompatibility.

◆ No safe level of alcohol consumption exists for pregnant women.

◆ Neonates with PKU require a diet low in phenylalanine.

◆ A cleft lip is surgically repaired several weeks after birth.

◆ Neonates with HIV infection initially may test falsely positive because of transplacental transfer of maternal HIV antibodies to the fetus; final diagnosis may take up to 6 months.

STUDY QUESTIONS

To evaluate your understanding of this chapter, answer the following questions in the space provided; then compare your responses with the correct answers in Appendix B, pages 174 and 175.

1. What is the pathophysiologic basis for transient tachypnea of the neonate?

_____

_____

2. When is RhoGAM ineffective? _____

_____

_____

3. What are the clinical manifestations of hydrocephaly? _____

_____

_____

4. What group of diseases is collectively known as TORCH? _____

_____

_____

CRITICAL THINKING AND APPLICATION EXERCISES

1. Observe a nurse working with high-risk neonates. Analyze the roles assumed and the functions associated with each role.

2. Prepare a drug card for AZT.

3. Create a patient-specific instruction sheet for the parents of a premature infant.

The Normal Postpartum Period

CHAPTER OVERVIEW

A new mother experiences many physiologic and psychological changes during the postpartum period. Knowledge of these changes is essential to guide appropriate nursing interventions. The nurse plays a key role in providing comprehensive postpartum teaching.

♦ I. Physiologic changes after pregnancy

A. Vascular system
   1. Decreased blood volume and increased hematocrit after vaginal delivery
   2. Extensive activation of blood clotting factors
   3. Return of blood volume to prenatal levels within 3 weeks

B. Reproductive system
   1. Rapid uterine INVOLUTION
   2. Cessation of progesterone production until first ovulation
   3. Permanent alteration of cervical external os shape from a circle to a jagged slit
   4. Endometrial regeneration within 6 weeks after delivery

C. Gastrointestinal system
   1. Delayed bowel movement from decreased intestinal muscle tone and perineal discomfort
   2. Increased thirst from fluids lost during labor and delivery
   3. Increased hunger after labor and delivery

D. Genitourinary system
   1. Increased urine output during the first 24 hours after delivery from puerperal diuresis
   2. Increased bladder capacity
   3. Proteinuria from the catalytic process of involution (in 50% of women)
   4. Decreased bladder-filling sensation from swelling and bruising of tissues
   5. Return of dilated ureters and renal pelvis to prepregnancy size by 6 weeks

E. Endocrine system
   1. Increased thyroid function
   2. Increased production of anterior pituitary gonadotropic hormones
   3. Decreased production of estrogen, aldosterone, progesterone, human chorionic gonadotropin, corticoids, and 17-ketosteroids

♦ II. Psychological changes after pregnancy

A. General information
   1. Mothers typically undergo psychological adjustments during the postpartum period
   2. Reva Rubin, a researcher who examined maternal adaptation to childbirth in the 1960s, identified three phases that can help the nurse understand maternal behavior after delivery

B. Phases
  1. Taking-in phase (maternal behavior 1 to 2 days after delivery)
    a. Is passive and dependent
    b. Directs energy towards herself instead of toward her infant
    c. May relive her labor and delivery to integrate the process into her life
    d. May find difficulty in making decisions
  2. Taking-hold phase (maternal behavior approximately 2 to 7 days after delivery)
    a. Has more energy
    b. Demonstrates independence and initiates self-care activities
    c. Accepts increasing responsibility for her neonate
    d. May be receptive to infant care and self-care education
    e. May express lack of confidence in caring for the infant
  3. Letting-go phase (maternal behavior approximately 7 days after delivery)
    a. Readjusts relationships with family members, such as assuming the mother role
    b. Assumes responsibility for her dependent neonate
    c. Recognizes the infant as separate from the self and relinquishes the fantasized infant
    d. May experience depression

◆ III. Neonate's impact on the family

A. Sibling reaction
  1. Siblings typically dislike the idea of sharing parents with the infant
  2. Reactions of siblings will depend on their age, the total number of siblings in the household, and the amount of preparation invested by the parents
  3. Regression is a normal reaction to the infant

B. Paternal reaction
  1. Fathers as well as mothers need to discuss the labor and delivery experience to integrate it into life experiences
  2. The father may feel left out when attention is given to the newborn and mother
  3. Fathers usually have less experience in and knowledge about infant care; thus, they need to be involved in the teaching plan

C. Mother-father relationship
  1. The time and effort devoted to infant care can strain the mother-father relationship
  2. The father may become jealous of the mother-infant bond
  3. The parents should consider babysitting arrangements to allow private time for themselves

◆ IV. Postpartum nursing care

A. Vital signs

1. Monitor vital signs every 4 hours for the first 24 hours and then every shift thereafter
2. The patient's temperature may be elevated to 100.4° F (38° C) from dehydration and exertion of labor
3. Blood pressure is usually normotensive within 24 hours of delivery
4. Bradycardia of 50 to 70 beats/minute is common during the first 6 to 10 days after delivery because of reductions in cardiac strain, stroke volume, and the vascular bed
5. The respiratory rate returns to normal after delivery

B. Fundus

1. Check the tone and location of the fundus (the uppermost portion of the uterus) every shift to assess involution

   a. The involuting uterus should be at the midline
   b. The fundus is usually midway between the umbilicus and symphysis 1 to 2 hours after delivery, 1 cm above or at the level of the umbilicus 12 hours after delivery, and about 3 cm below the umbilicus by the third day after delivery
   c. The fundus will continue to descend about 1 cm/day until it is not palpable above the symphysis (about 9 days after delivery); the uterus decreases to its prepregnancy size 5 to 6 weeks after delivery, not from a decrease in the number of cells but from a decrease in their size
   d. The fundus should feel firm to the touch

2. A firm uterus helps control postpartum hemorrhage by clamping down on uterine blood vessels
3. A boggy (soft) fundus should be massaged gently; if the fundus does not respond, a firmer touch should be used
4. The doctor may prescribe oxytocin (Pitocin), ergonovine maleate (Ergotrate Maleate), or methylergonovine maleate (Methergine) to maintain uterine firmness

CLINICAL ALERT

5. The uterus may relax if overstimulated by massage or medications
6. A distended bladder can impede the downward descent of the uterus by pushing it upward and possibly to the side; the nurse should suspect a distended bladder if the uterus is not firm at the midline
7. Any vaginal bleeding that is considered excessive should be evaluated (See *Intervening with excessive vaginal bleeding,* page 138)
8. A multipara is more prone to "after-pains" from uterine contractions; "after-pains" generally last 2 to 3 days and may be intensified by breast-feeding

C. Lochia

1. Assess LOCHIA (discharge after delivery from sloughing of the uterine decidua) during every shift, noting its color, amount, odor, and consistency

   a. Lochia rubra is the vaginal discharge for the first 3 days after delivery; it has a fleshy odor and is bloody with small clots

   b. Lochia serosa refers to the vaginal discharge during days 4 to 9; it is pinkish or brown with a serosanguineous consistency and fleshy odor

   c. Lochia alba is a yellow to white discharge that usually begins about 10 days after delivery; it may last from 2 to 6 weeks

CLINICAL ALERT

2. Foul-smelling lochia may indicate an infection

3. Continuous seepage of bright red blood may indicate a cervical or vaginal laceration; additional evaluation is necessary

   a. Lochia that saturates a sanitary pad within 45 minutes usually indicates an abnormally heavy flow

   b. Lochial discharge may diminish after a cesarean delivery

4. A heavier flow of lochia may occur when the patient first rises from bed because of pooling of the lochia in the vagina

5. Numerous large clots should be evaluated further; they may interfere with involution

6. Breast-feeding and exertion may increase lochial flow

7. Lochia may be scant but should never be absent; this may indicate a postpartum infection

D. Breasts

1. Assess the size and shape of the patient's breasts every shift, noting reddened areas, tenderness, or engorgement

2. Check the nipples for cracking, fissures, or soreness

3. Advise the patient to wear a support bra to maintain shape and enhance comfort

E. Elimination

CLINICAL ALERT

1. Assess the patient's elimination patterns

2. The patient should void within the first 6 to 8 hours after delivery

   a. The nurse should assess for a distended bladder within the first few hours after delivery; a distended bladder can interfere with uterine involution

   b. The patient may use pain medication before urination or pour warm water over the perineum to eliminate the fear of pain

   c. The patient who cannot void may require catheterization

3. The patient should be encouraged to have a bowel movement within 1 or 2 days after delivery to avoid constipation

DECISION TREE
Intervening with excessive vaginal bleeding

Use the decision tree below to help guide your interventions when you determine that your patient has excessive vaginal bleeding.

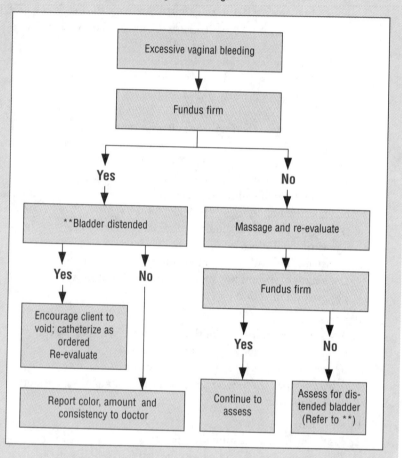

a. The nurse should encourage increased fluid and roughage intake and alleviate maternal anxieties regarding pain from or damage to the episiotomy site

b. The patient may require laxatives, stool softeners, suppositories, or enemas

c. A patient with a fourth-degree laceration should never be given anything rectally

F. Episiotomy
1. Assess the episiotomy site every shift to evaluate healing, noting erythema, intactness of stitches, edema, and any odor or drainage
2. The edges of an episiotomy are usually sealed 24 hours after delivery
   a. The patient with a mediolateral episiotomy can be positioned on that side to provide better visibility and less discomfort
   b. The patient with a midline episiotomy may be positioned on the side or the back during assessment

G. Rectal area
1. Assess the rectal area
2. Note the number and appearance of hemorrhoids

H. Medications
1. Administer medications to relieve discomfort from the episiotomy, uterine contractions, incisional pain, or engorged breasts, as prescribed
   a. Analgesics include propoxyphene (Darvocet-N), acetaminophen, aspirin, oxycodone with acetaminophen (Percocet), butalbital with aspirin (Fiorinal), ibuprophin (Motrin) and codeine
   b. Stool softeners and laxatives include docusate calcium (Surfak), docusate sodium (Colace), and magnesium hydroxide (milk of magnesia)
   c. Oxytocic agents, such as methylergonovine maleate (Methergine), oxytocin (Pitocin), and ergonovine maleate (Ergotrate maleate), help prevent or treat postpartum hemorrhage
   d. Bromocriptine mesylate (Parlodel) may be ordered to help suppress lactation
2. Monitor for therapeutic effect

◆ **V. Postpartum patient teaching**

A. Self-care instructions to the mother
1. Personal hygiene
   a. Change perineal pads frequently, removing from front to back
   b. Immediately report lochia with a foul smell, heavy flow, or clots
   c. Take a sitz bath three to four times daily
   d. Take a daily shower to relieve discomfort of normal postpartum diaphoresis
   e. Dispose of perineal pads in plastic bag
2. Sexual activity and contraception
   a. Follow the doctor's instructions on sexual activity and contraception
      (1) Most couples can resume sexual activity within 3 to 4 weeks after delivery
      (2) Breast-feeding is not a reliable form of contraception

(3) About 50% of bottle-feeding mothers ovulate during the first cycle after delivery; about 80% of breast-feeding mothers have several anovulatory cycles before ovulating

b. Use a water-based lubricant, if needed (steroid depletion may diminish vaginal lubrication for up to 6 months)

c. Expect decreased intensity and rapidity of sexual response (a normal response for about 3 months after delivery)

d. Perform Kegel exercises to help strengthen the pubococcygeal muscles

3. Weight loss

a. Expect to lose about 5 lb (2.2 kg) from diuresis during the early PUERPERIUM (in addition to the 10 to 12 lb [4.5 to 5.4 kg] typically lost after delivery)

b. Expect to return to prepregnancy weight within 6 to 8 weeks after delivery (if weight gain during pregnancy was 25 to 30 lb [11.3 to 13.6 kg])

4. Activity and exercise

a. Request assistance in getting out of bed the first several times after delivery to minimize dizziness and fainting from medications, blood loss, and decreased food intake

b. Begin exercising when the doctor permits it

c. Sit with the legs elevated for about 30 minutes if lochia increases or lochia rubra returns, either of which may indicate excessive activity; if excessive vaginal discharge persists, notify the doctor

d. Expect abdominal muscle tone to increase within 2 to 3 months after delivery

5. Nutrition

a. Increase protein and caloric intake to restore body tissues (if breast-feeding, increase daily caloric intake by 200 kcal over the pregnancy requirement of 2,400 kcal)

b. Expect increased thirst because of postpartum diuresis

6. Comfort measures

a. To relieve perineal discomfort, use ice packs (for the first 8 to 12 hours to minimize edema); spray peri bottles; sitz baths; anesthetic sprays, creams, and pads (such as witch hazel pads); and prescribed pain medications

b. To relieve discomfort from engorged breasts, wear a support bra or binder, apply ice packs, and take prescribed medications; if breast-feeding, eat frequent meals, apply warm compresses, and express milk manually

7. Psychosocial adjustments

a. Don't be alarmed by mood swings and bouts of depression; these are normal postpartum responses

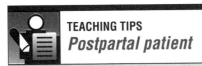

TEACHING TIPS
Postpartal patient

Be sure to include the following topic areas in your teaching plan for your postpartal patient:
- Physiologic and psychosocial changes
- Lochial changes to report
- Breast care
- Activity and exercise
- Nutrition and diet
- Comfort measures
- Care of the neonate
- Signs and symptoms to report to doctor
- Contraceptive methods if desired

      (1) More than half of postpartum women experience transient mood alterations called "baby blues"
      (2) Common signs and symptoms include sadness, crying, fatigue, and low self-esteem
      (3) Possible causes include hormonal changes, genetic predisposition, and altered role and self-concept
   b. Know that mood swings typically occur within the first 3 weeks after delivery and usually subside within 1 to 10 days

B. Neonate care instructions to the parents
  1. Cord care
    a. Wipe the umbilical cord with alcohol, especially around the base, at every diaper change
    b. Report promptly any odor, discharge, or signs of skin irritation around the cord
    c. Fold the diaper below the cord until the cord falls off (about 7 to 10 days)
  2. Circumcised penis
    a. Gently clean the penis with water and apply fresh petroleum gauze with each diaper change
    b. Loosen petroleum gauze stuck to the penis by pouring warm water over the area
    c. Do not remove yellow discharge that covers the glans about 24 hours after circumcision; this is part of normal healing
    d. Report promptly any foul-smelling, purulent discharge
    e. Apply diapers loosely until the circumcision heals (about 5 days)

CLINICAL ALERT
  3. Uncircumcised penis
    a. Do not retract the foreskin when washing the infant because the foreskin is adhered to the glans

b. Understand that natural loosening of the foreskin begins at birth; however, it is retractable in only about 50% of males age 1

4. Elimination

a. Become familiar with the infant's voiding patterns (usually six to eight wet diapers daily)

b. Become familiar with the infant's bowel patterns (usually two to three stools daily; more frequently if breast-fed)

(1) The first stool is called meconium; it is an odorless, dark-green, thick substance containing bile, fetal epithelial cells, and hair

(2) Transitional stools occur approximately 2 to 3 days after in-gestion of milk; they are greenish-brown and thinner than meconium

(3) The stool changes to a pasty, yellow, pungent stool (bottle-fed infant) or to a sweet-smelling loose yellow stool (breast-fed infant) by the fourth day

5. Thermometer use

a. Insert a lubricated thermometer into the rectum for 4 to 5 min-utes, or carefully place an axillary thermometer under the arm and hold in place for 10 minutes

b. Be aware of alternate devices including a plastic temperature strip, pacifiers with thermometer built in or tympanic ther-mometers.

6. Diapering

a. Change diapers before and after every feeding

b. Avoid diaper rash by frequent diaper changes and thorough cleaning and drying of the skin

c. Expose the infant's buttocks to the air and light several times a day for approximately 20 minutes to treat diaper rash; apply ointment to minimize contact with urine and feces

d. Do not use ointments and powders together; they will cake on the skin and further irritate it

CLINICAL ALERT

7. Bathing

a. Give the infant sponge baths until the cord falls off; then wash the infant in a tub containing 3″ to 4″ (7.6 to 10 cm) of warm water

b. Place a washcloth on the bottom of the tub or sink to prevent slipping

c. Avoid using perfumed or deodorant soap

d. Organize supplies before the bath to avoid interruptions

e. Avoid drafts

f. Clean the eye from the inner to outer canthus with plain water

g. Vary the frequency of bathing with weather; a bath every other day during winter is sufficient

8. Clothing
   a. Dress the infant appropriately according to indoor temperatures and outdoor weather conditions
   b. Provide the infant with a hat to avoid drafts and minimize heat loss through the scalp when outdoors
9. Breast-feeding (see also *Physiology of lactation,* page 145)
   a. Initiate breast-feeding as soon as possible after delivery and then feed the infant on demand
      (1) Expect about 90% of breast milk to be emptied from the breasts within the first 7 minutes of feeding
      (2) Position the infant's mouth slightly differently at each feeding to reduce irritation at one site
      (3) Burp the infant before switching to the other breast
      (4) Insert the little finger into a corner of the baby's mouth to separate the baby from the nipple
      (5) Experiment with various breast-feeding positions (cradle, football hold, side-lying, and Australian or back-lying) to find the most comfortable one
   b. Perform thorough breast care to promote cleanliness and comfort
      (1) After each feeding, wash the nipples and areolae with plain warm water and air dry during the first 2 to 3 weeks to prevent nipple soreness; after that, daily washing is adequate for cleanliness
      (2) Avoid using soap, which can dry and crack the nipples and leave an undesirable taste for the infant
      (3) Apply nonalcohol cream to the nipple and areola to prevent drying and cracking
      (4) Wear a well-fitted nursing bra that provides support and contains flaps that can be loosened easily before feeding
      (5) Use breast pads to avoid staining clothes from leakage, and change wet pads promptly to avoid skin breakdown
      (6) Empty engorged breasts manually or with a breast pump
         (a) Expressed breast milk can be placed in a sterile bottle and stored in the refrigerator for 24 hours
         (b) Expressed breast milk can be frozen for up to 4 months
   c. Follow a diet that ensures adequate nutrition for the mother and infant
      (1) Drink at least four 8-oz glasses of fluid daily
      (2) Increase daily caloric intake by 200 kcal over the pregnancy requirement of 2,400 kcal
      (3) Know that ingested substances (caffeine, alcohol, and medications) can pass into breast milk

      (4) Avoid foods that cause irritability, gas, or diarrhea

  d. Consult the pediatrician before taking any medication

  e. Consider joining a breast-feeding support group, if desired

10. Formula preparation and feeding

  a. Follow the pediatrician's instructions

  b. Investigate various forms of formula available (ready-to-feed, concentrated, and powder) and preparation methods

  c. Feed the infant in an upright position, and keep the nipple full of formula to minimize air swallowing

  d. Burp the infant after each ounce of formula (more frequently if the infant spits up); hold the infant upright against the shoulder for burping

    (1) Holding the infant across the lap for burping may bring up milk along with the air

    (2) Holding the infant in a sitting position may prove ineffective because the air cannot easily exit the stomach

    (3) An infant who has not burped after 3 minutes of gentle patting and rubbing may not need to burp

11. Handling

  a. Be aware that infants have an inborn fear of falling and become upset if left unsupported or if their position is abruptly changed

  b. Do not startle the infant; talk softly and touch gently before picking the infant up

  c. Support the infant's head; the infant cannot control it

12. Health promotion and illness prevention

  a. Do not expose the infant to persons with communicable illnesses

  b. Minimize the infant's exposure to crowds

  c. Provide adequate covering and clothing

  d. Use a reliable car seat (legally required)

  e. Immediately report signs and symptoms of illness to the pediatrician

    (1) Temperature greater than 101° F (38.3° C) or below 97° F (36.1° C)

    (2) Projectile vomiting

    (3) Lethargy

    (4) Cyanosis

    (5) Change in normal feeding pattern

    (6) Change in normal elimination pattern

Physiology of lactation

Milk is produced in the breast alveoli, tiny sacs made up of epithelial cells. The female breast has a rich blood supply from which the alveoli extract nutrients to produce milk. The alveoli are situated in lobules, clusters leading to ductules that merge into lactiferous ducts; these larger ducts widen further into ampullae or lactiferous sinuses located behind the nipple and areola.

Lactation is controlled by hormone secretion from numerous endocrine glands, particularly the pituitary hormones prolactin and oxytocin. Factors involved in establishing and maintaining lactation include the anatomic structure of the mammary gland; the development of alveoli, ducts, and nipples; initiation and maintenance of milk secretion; and ejection or propulsion of milk from the alveoli to the nipple. Lactation also is influenced by the suckling process and by maternal emotions.

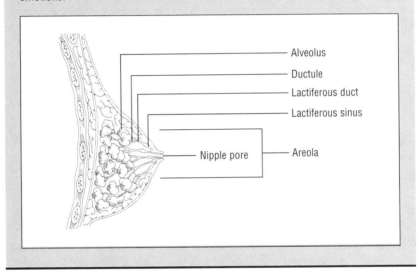

POINTS TO REMEMBER

♦ The postpartum period is marked by complex psychological and physiologic adjustments.

♦ The addition of a newborn to a family will affect all of its members.

♦ Overstimulation of the uterus may result in uterine relaxation with subsequent excessive blood loss.

♦ Subinvolution of the uterus can lead to postpartum hemorrhage.

◆ Postpartal nursing care focuses on vital signs, fundus (uterine involution), lochia, breasts, elimination, episiotomy, rectal area, adminstration of medications, if ordered, and patient teaching.

STUDY QUESTIONS

To evaluate your understanding of this chapter, answer the following questions in the space provided; then compare your responses with the correct answers in Appendix B, page 175.

1. What should a new mother anticipate about her urine output in the first 24 hours after delivery? _____

_____

_____

2. What are the three phases of psychological adjustment during the postpartum period? _____

_____

_____

3. How can a distended bladder affect the uterus? _____

_____

_____

4. Describe how lochia changes within the first few weeks following delivery.

_____

_____

5. How many calories should a breast-feeding mother consume daily? _____

_____

_____

6. What should the nurse teach parents about the neonate's cord care? _____

_____

_____

7. How should a breast-feeding mother care for her nipples? _____

_____

_____

CRITICAL THINKING AND APPLICATION EXERCISES

1. Prepare a class demonstration on how to bathe a neonate properly.

2. Develop drug cards for ergonovine maleate, methylergonovine maleate, and bromocriptine mesylate.

3. Create a patient-specific instruction sheet for a postpartum patient planning to breast-feed.

4. Follow a postpartum patient from admission to the unit through discharge. Develop a patient-specific plan of care, including any needs for follow-up and education.

11

Complications and High-Risk Conditions of the Postpartum Period

CHAPTER OVERVIEW

During the postpartum period, women remain at risk for complications due to many factors, including fatigue, blood loss, trauma, and infection. Prevention or early detection is vital to minimize difficulties during this period of great physiologic and psychological stress. The patient with human immunodeficiency virus (HIV) needs special attention throughout the pregnancy, but especially during the postpartal period.

◆ I. Mastitis

A. General information
1. Inflammation of the breast
2. Seen primarily in breast-feeding patients
3. Causative organism usually is *Staphylococcus aureus* from the newborn's throat or nose, from hospital personnel, or from the mother

B. Clinical manifestations
1. Temperature is elevated
2. Breast is red, warm, and tender; usually appearing 2 to 4 weeks after delivery
3. Mastitis is usually unilateral and breast milk may become scant

C. Prevention
1. Encourage frequent breast-feeding
   Instruct in thorough handwashing
3. Demonstrate how to manually release blocked milk ducts

D. Management
1. Administration of antibiotics and analgesics
2. Application of local heat
3. Possible cessation of breast-feeding (medical opinions vary concerning continuation or stoppage of breast-feeding during the acute phase)
4. Patient education (For teaching tips, see *Patient with mastitis,* page 150)

◆ II. Late postpartum hemorrhage

A. General information
1. Blood loss of more than 500 ml later than 24 hours after delivery
2. Sometimes not occurring until 5 to 15 days after delivery
3. Predisposing factors:
   a. Delivery of a large infant
   b. Hydramnios
   c. Dystocia
   d. Grand multiparity
   e. Trauma during delivery

B. Etiology
1. Uterine atony
2. Incomplete placental separation
3. Laceration of the birth canal
4. Retained placental fragments

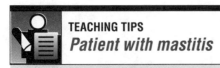

TEACHING TIPS
Patient with mastitis

Be sure to include the following topics in your teaching plan for the patient with mastitis:
- Underlying cause of mastitis
- Hand-washing procedure
- Heat application, including technique, frequency, and duration
- Breast emptying techniques, if breast-feeding
- Medication regimen
- Follow-up

    C. Management
        1. Careful assessment of uterine tone
           Assessment of color, amount, and consistency of lochia
        3. Monitoring of vital signs
        4. Maintenance of a pad count
        5. Administration of oxytocics

◆ III. SUBINVOLUTION of the uterus

    A. General information
        1. Failure of the uterus to return to its normal size after childbirth
        2. Diagnosis usually made at the postpartum checkup, 4 to 6 weeks after delivery
        3. Predisposing factors: retained placental fragments and infection

    B. Clinical manifestations
        1. Displacement of the uterus in the abdominal cavity
        2. Persistent lochia rubra, leukorrhea, and backache

    C. Management
        1. Administration of oxytocins and antibiotics
        2. Possible dilatation and curettage

◆ IV. Puerperal psychiatric disorders

    A. General information
        1. Puerperal psychiatric disorders include depression, mania, schizophrenia, and psychosis
        2. These occur in 1% to 2% of all normal childbirths

    B. Depression
        1. The most common disorder
        2. Peaks approximately 6 weeks after delivery

3. Clinical manifestations (may last up to several months)
   a. Suicidal thinking
   b. Feelings of failure
   c. Exhaustion
4. Management
   a. Psychotherapy
   b. Medications, commonly a tranquilizer with a prominent stimulating effect

C. Mania
   1. May occur 1 to 2 weeks after delivery
   2. Sometimes occurring after a brief period of depression
   3. Clinical manifestations
      a. Agitation
      b. Excitement that may last 1 to 3 weeks
   4. Management
      a. Psychotherapy
      b. Medication, commonly a tranquilizer with a prominent sedative effect

D. Schizophrenia
   1. May appear by the 10th day after delivery
   2. Clinical manifestations
      a. Delusional thinking
      b. Gross distortion of reality
      c. Flight of ideas
      d. Possible rejection of the father, infant, or both
   3. Management
      a. Phenothiazine administration
      b. Psychotherapy
      c. Possible hospitalization

E. Psychosis
   1. Can appear from 2 weeks to 12 months after delivery
   2. Clinical manifestations
      a. Sleep disturbances
      b. Restlessness
      c. Depression
      d. Indecisiveness progressing to bewilderment, perplexity, a dreamy state, impaired memory, confusion, and somatic delusion
   3. Management
      a. Medication
      b. Psychotherapy
      c. Possible hospitalization

◆ V. HEMATOMA

A. General information
1. Collection of blood (25 to 500 ml) in the soft tissue
2. Most commonly seen in the vulva and vagina
3. Related to vascular injury during a spontaneous or assisted delivery

**CLINICAL
ALERT**

B. Clinical manifestations
1. Severe vulvar pain (requires immediate investigation to rule out hematoma)
2. Unilateral purplish discoloration of the perineum and buttocks, which are firm and tender
3. Feeling of fullness in the vagina

C. Management
1. Application of small ice packs
2. Surgical evacuation

◆ VI. Puerperal infection

A. General information
1. Postpartum infection of the reproductive tract that may remain localized (endometritis, salpingitis) or extend to other parts of the body (peritonitis, pelvic cellulitis)
2. Caused by introduction of vaginal microorganisms into the sterile uterine cavity via premature rupture of membranes, operative incisions, hematomas, damaged tissues, or lapses in aseptic technique

B. Clinical manifestations (depend on the site and extent of infection)
1. Foul-smelling lochia
2. Lethargy
3. Abdominal pain

**CLINICAL
ALERT**

4. Subinvolution of the uterus
5. Sustained fever of at least 100.4° F (38° C)

C. Management
1. Antibiotic therapy
2. Sitz baths
3. Positioning to enhance drainage
4. Maintenance of fluid and electrolyte balance

**CLINICAL
ALERT**

5. Monitoring of vital signs and symptoms
6. Because a large percentage of postpartum morbidity results from infection, the Joint Committee on Maternal Welfare issued the following definition of puerperal morbidity: "Temperature of 100.4° F (38° C) or above, the temperature to occur on any two of the first 10 postpartum days, exclusive of the first 24 hours and to be taken by mouth by a standard technique at least four times a day."

◆ VII. The patient with acquired immunodeficiency syndrome (AIDS)

A. General information

1. Life-threatening disease caused by the human immunodeficiency virus (HIV) in which the body's immune system becomes susceptible to opportunistic infections

2. An illness characterized by laboratory evidence of HIV infection co-existing with one or more indicator diseases, such as herpes simplex cytomegalovirus, *Pneumocystis carinii,* Kaposi's sarcoma, wasting syndrome

B. Women at risk

1. I.V. drug users
2. Those with multiple sex partners
3. Recipients of contaminated blood or blood products
4. Partners of those considered high risk

C. Pathophysiology

1. HIV, a retrovirus, selectively infects human cells containing a CD4 antigen on their surface, the majority of which are T4 lymphocytes
2. HIV infects the T4 cells and when stimulated, HIV is rapidly produced, destroying and killing the T4 cells.
3. HIV infection renders the patient immunodeficient and predisposes the patient to opportunistic infections, unusual cancers, and other characteristic abnormalities

D. Management

1. For prenatal and intrapartal management, see *Patient with AIDS: Prenatal and intrapartal management,* page 154

2. Postpartal management

   a. It is best to avoid circumcision if mother is HIV-positive
   b. Follow-up care for both infant and mother should be arranged prior to discharge
   c. Discuss birth control alternatives before discharge; intrauterine devices should be avoided — a barrier method, such as a condom, is the best choice
   d. Maintain standard body fluid precautions
      (1) Wear disposable gloves and a plastic apron when in direct contact with the patient's blood or body fluids (specimens, dressings, excretions, linen, trash, amniotic fluid, and sanitary pads)
      (2) Dispose of contaminated needles and syringes in a puncture-resistant receptacle in the patient's room
      (3) Double-bag trash and linen before removing from the room

Patient with AIDS: Prenatal and intrapartal management

The chart below focuses on managing the patient with AIDS (acquired immunodeficiency syndrome) during the prenatal and intrapartal periods. Special emphasis is given to AZT therapy.

	MANAGEMENT	A.Z.T. PROPHYLAXIS CRITERIA
Prenatal period	• Pneumococcal vaccine • Bactrim prophylaxis if CD4$^+$ count < 200/μl • Avoidance of amniocentesis and PUBS • Ultrasound for growth every 4 weeks • Thorough physical examination and counseling • Laboratory studies, including gonorrhea and *Chlamydia* cultures, PPD and anergy panel, and serologies	• Greater than 14 weeks' gestation • Patient has not received AZT for more than 6 months in the past • Baseline CD4$^+$ counts > 200/μl • AZT prophylaxis 200 mg P.O. t.i.d. • Although use of AZT during prenatal period has decreased the maternal-fetal transmission rate of human immunodeficiency virus from 25% to 8%, the patient must be counseled about unknown long-term risks
Intrapartal period	• Avoidance of scalp sampling and scalp electrodes, if possible • Scalp stimulation may be a satisfactory alternative	• AZT prophylaxis: 2 mg/kg I.V. loading dose, followed by 1 mg/kg/hr until delivery

    (4) Place laboratory specimens in a plastic bag before removing from the room

E. Psychosocial considerations
1. Psychological implications emerge from the probable low survival rate of the mother and her child
2. Direct mother-infant contact should not be avoided unless open skin lesions are involved

CLINICAL ALERT

3. Strict isolation is necessary only if the patient has tuberculosis, open lesions, or copious secretions or blood
4. Breast-feeding is contraindicated because HIV can be transmitted via breast milk

POINTS TO REMEMBER

◆ A late postpartum hemorrhage may not occur until 5 to 15 days after delivery.

◆ Subinvolution of the uterus may result from retained placental fragments and infections.

◆ Puerperal psychosis may take up to 12 months following delivery to appear.

◆ HIV can be transmitted via breast milk.

STUDY QUESTIONS

To evaluate your understanding of this chapter, answer the following questions in the space provided; then compare your responses with the correct answers in Appendix B, page 175.

1. What is the causative organism of mastitis and its most common sources?

   _____

   _____

2. What predisposing factors identify the patient at increased risk for a late postpartum hemorrhage? _____

   _____

   _____

3. What are the clinical manifestations of a vulva or vaginal hematoma?_____

   _____

   _____

4. What should nursing management of the HIV-positive patient include during the postpartum period? _____

   _____

   _____

CRITICAL THINKING AND APPLICATION EXERCISES

1. Develop a chart comparing early and late postpartal hemorrhage, including predisposing factors, etiology, manifestations, and management.

2. Observe a dilatation and curettage performed on a patient with uterine subinvolution. Prepare a class presentation for your fellow classmates describing the nursing care before, during, and after the procedure.

3. Follow a patient with a postpartal complication from admission through discharge. Develop a patient-specific plan of care, including any needs for follow-up and education.

Reproductive Issues and Concerns

LEARNING OBJECTIVES

After studying this chapter, you should be able to:

♦ Identify the basic principles of genetics, common screening and diagnostic techniques, and patients who require genetic counseling, screening, and testing.

♦ State the nurse's role in caring for the family with a possible genetic disorder.

♦ Identify the goals of family planning. Describe how various methods of contraception prevent pregnancy. Discuss the nurse's role in family planning.

♦ Describe various emotional responses to an elective abortion. Discuss methods of pregnancy termination during each trimester.

♦ Describe possible male and female causes of infertility and diagnostic tests used to determine the cause.

♦ Identify the emotional reactions that a couple may experience in coping with infertility.

♦ Describe surgical and nonsurgical methods of treating infertility and other options for the infertile couple.

CHAPTER OVERVIEW

A woman's ability to reproduce carries with it many choices and uncertainties. Many of these choices involve emotional issues with ethical and legal implications. The nurse plays a key role, providing accurate information to allow patients to make an informed decision and supporting the patients nonjudgmentally.

♦ I. Genetic disorders

A. General information

1. Genetic information is stored on chromosomes, tightly coiled strands of deoxyribonucleic acid (DNA)
2. Chromosomes are composed of DNA, histone proteins, and nonhistone proteins
3. Chromosomes contain thousands of genes; these are the smallest units of hereditary information, lined up in a specific pattern
4. The normal number of chromosomes is 46: 22 pairs of autosomes and one pair of sex chromosomes (XX for female and XY for male)
5. A pictorial analysis of chromosomes (karyotype) can be performed most easily on the lymphocytes, but also on skin, bone marrow, or organ tissue
6. A genetic disorder can be classified as CONGENITAL or HEREDITARY

B. Mendel's laws

1. Principle of dominance
   a. Genes are not equal in strength
   b. The stronger gene, producing an observable trait, is called *dominant*
   c. The weaker gene, whose trait is not seen, is called *recessive*
2. Principle of segregation
   a. Paired chromosomes that contain genes from both parents separate during meiosis
   b. Chance determines whether the maternal or paternal gene travels to a specific gamete
3. Principle of independent assortment: pairs of genes are distributed in the gametes in random fashion, unrelated to any other pairs

C. Categories of genetic disorders

1. Single gene
   a. Traits are determined by two genes, one from each parent
      (1) Autosomal traits are determined by a gene on an autosome

(2) Sex-linked traits are determined by a gene on a sex chromosome

b. The disease trait in autosomal-dominant inheritance disorders is HETEROZYGOUS

(1) These disorders are caused by an abnormal dominant gene on an autosome

(2) These include Marfan's syndrome, osteogenesis imperfecta, and Huntington's disease

c. The disease trait in autosomal-recessive inheritance disorders is HOMOZYGOUS

(1) The normal gene is dominant, so the individual must have two abnormal genes to be affected

(2) Examples include sickle-cell anemia, Tay-Sachs disease, cystic fibrosis, and most metabolic diseases

d. The abnormal gene in X-linked recessive inheritance disorders is carried on the X chromosome; examples include hemophilia, Duchenne's disease (pseudohypertrophic muscular dystrophy), and color blindness

e. X-linked dominant inheritance disorders are similar to X-linked recessive disorders, except that heterozygous females are affected

(1) Occurrence is rare

(2) An example is vitamin D-resistant rickets

2. Chromosomal ABERRATIONS (deviations in either the number or structure of chromosomes)

a. A structural defect can be caused by a loss, addition, or rearrangement of the genes on a chromosome or by the exchange of genes between chromosomes

b. Deviations in the number of chromosomes involve either the gain or loss of an entire chromosome during cell division; the suffix *-somy* is used in disorders with abnormal numbers

c. Nondisjunction is the failure of chromosomes to separate during cell division

d. Translocation is the joining of two chromosomes to make one larger double chromosome

e. The most common chromosomal disorder is Down syndrome (trisomy 21)

3. Multifactorial inheritance disorders

a. Two types of multifactorial inheritance disorders exist

(1) In the first type, genes and the environment interact to produce an aberration

(2) In the second type, no inheritance pattern is identifiable, but risk of recurrence is higher in certain families

b. Examples include cleft lip and palate, congenital dislocated hip, congenital heart defects, neural tube defects, and pyloric stenosis

    D. Detection of genetic disorders

        1. Indications for preconception genetic counseling

            a. Members of a high-risk group (for example, Tay-Sachs disease among Ashkenazic Jews)

            b. Members of families with a history of genetic disorders

        2. Indications for prenatal genetic testing

            a. Pregnant patient age 35 or older

            b. Couple who previously produced a child with a genetic disorder

            c. Couple that is heterozygous for a recessive disorder

            d. Couple in which one or both partners have a genetic disorder

            e. Female who is a carrier of an X-linked disorder

        3. Prenatal testing methods

            a. Amniocentesis (see Chapter 4, The Normal Prenatal Period, for more information)

            b. Ultrasonography: detects anencephaly, microcephaly, and hydrocephaly

            c. Roentgenography: detects bone abnormalities

        4. Postdelivery detection

            a. Biochemical tests for phenylketonuria, hypothyroidism, and galactosemia

            b. Cytologic studies for an infant whose appearance suggests a chromosomal aberration

            c. Dermatoglyphics to determine chromosomal aberrations by evaluating dermal ridges

    E. Nursing implications

        1. Understand genetic theory well enough to reinforce information given by the genetic counselor

CLINICAL ALERT

        2. Be aware of factors necessitating genetic counseling, such as increased age and family history when obtaining medical and obstetric history

        3. Prepare the patient by explaining the purpose of and procedure for each diagnostic test

        4. Assist with diagnostic testing as necessary

        5. Provide emotional support to those receiving genetic counseling

        6. Act as an advocate, counselor, and teacher; with advanced preparation and certification, the nurse can function as a genetic counselor

        7. Anticipate common responses to diagnoses of genetic disorders, such as apathy, denial, anger, hostility, fear, embarrassment, grief, and lowered self-esteem

◆ II. Family planning

A. General information

1. Family planning is a very personal topic that has many ethical, physical, emotional, religious, and legal implications
2. Through family planning, the couple is able to prevent unwanted pregnancies or control the timing and spacing of planned pregnancies

B. Methods

1. Mechanical barrier methods
   a. Methods that block the sperm from coming in contact with the ovum
   b. Examples: condoms, diaphragms, cervical cap
2. Hormonal contraceptives
   a. Methods that interfere with ovulation or implantation by altering hormone levels
   b. Examples: oral contraceptives, Depo-Provera, NORPLANT, the morning-after pill
3. Chemical barrier methods
   a. Methods that contain a spermicidal agent
   b. Examples: vaginal spermicide, vaginal contraceptive film
4. Natural methods
   a. Methods that help the woman identify physical signs and symptoms indicating ovulation and fertile periods
   b. Examples: rhythm method, basal body temperature, cervical mucus method, symptothermal method
5. Intrauterine devices: insertion of device into the uterus that prevents implantation of a fertilized ovum by altering the surface of the endometrium
6. Coitus interruptus: withdrawal of the penis from the vagina prior to ejaculation

C. Nursing implications

1. Carefully evaluate own personal beliefs and attitudes regarding family planning and provide open, nonjudgmental counseling in a trusting setting
2. If possible, include the male in teaching sessions
3. Include in discussions about family planning information regarding prevention and treatment of sexually transmitted diseases (For teaching tips, see *Couple considering family planning,* page 162)
4. Play different roles including that of a teacher, counselor, advocate and researcher
   a. As a teacher, present information regarding various contraceptive methods as well as proper use

TEACHING TIPS
Couple considering family planning

Be sure to include the following topics in your teaching plan for the couple who is considering family planning:
- Underlying reasons for family planning
- Any physical, emotional, religious, or ethical concerns about family planning
- Contraceptive methods available
- Advantages and disadvantages of each
- Information about sexually transmitted diseases

    b. As a counselor, assist the woman in selecting the method that best suits her lifestyle and needs

    c. As advocate, support the woman's choice, regardless of personal beliefs

    d. As a researcher, participate in studies and identify new avenues to be evaluated

♦ III. Elective abortion

A. General information
1. Elective abortion refers to the willful termination of a pregnancy by mechanical or medical methods prior to the age of viability
2. Though legally permitted, elected abortions remain a highly charged religious and social subject
3. Different states have varying restrictions on timing, legality, counseling, and payment
4. Women also experience varying emotional responses
    a. While some women may be relieved the pregnancy is terminated, many women feel guilt or remorse
    b. Some women relive the experience each year on the anniversary of the abortion
    c. Some women report imagining what their lost child would look or act like when they see other children

B. Methods
1. Dilatation and evacuation
    a. Used in the first trimester
    b. Cervix is dilated by mechanical means
    c. Products of conception are removed by suction
2. Prostaglandin suppositories
    a. Used in the second and third trimesters
    b. Prostaglandin is inserted into the cervix, which causes dilation and initiation of contractions

C. Nursing implications
1. A nurse must carefully explore her own personal and religious beliefs regarding abortion; she can refuse to participate in an elective abortion because of moral or religious convictions
2. The nurse must present a nonjudgmental attitude when caring for the woman
3. The patient must be told she may experience grieving and a sense of loss

◆ IV. Infertility

A. General information
1. Defined as the inability to conceive after 1 year of consistent attempts without using contraceptives
2. Affects 15 to 20% of the couples in the U.S.

B. Types
1. Primary infertility
   a. The man has never impregnated a woman
   b. The woman has never been pregnant, despite consistent attempts to do so
2. Secondary infertility: the woman cannot conceive or sustain a pregnancy after an initial pregnancy
3. Sterility: an absolute factor (male or female) prevents pregnancy

C. Possible factors causing infertility
1. Female factors
   a. Endocrine disorders
   b. Genital tract obstruction
   c. Anatomic abnormalities (cervical, tubal, vaginal, uterine, or ovarian)
   d. Emotional disorder
   e. Preexisting medical condition
   f. Severe nutritional deficit
2. Male factors
   a. Genital tract obstruction
   b. Spermatozoal difficulties (reduced spermatozoa count, decreased motility, malformed spermatozoa)
   c. Abnormal genital tract secretions
   d. Coital difficulties (for instance, failure to deposit sperm at the cervix, which may be linked to obesity)
   e. Testicular abnormalities from illness, CRYPTORCHIDISM, trauma, or irradiation

D. Diagnostic measures
　1. Female
　　a. Menstrual, medical, fertility, sexual, surgical, and occupational history
　　b. Physical examination
　　c. Review of personal habits, including medications, use of tobacco and alcohol, exercise, weight history, and use of douches or vaginal deodorants
　　d. Laboratory examinations: complete blood count, sedimentation rate, serology, urinalysis, thyroid function tests, glucose tolerance tests, and hormonal testing, such as prolactin, adrenal, luteinizing hormone (LH), and follicle-stimulating hormone (FSH)
　　e. Cervical mucosal tests to assess elasticity and content
　　f. Postcoital sperm analysis to assess sperm mobility and morphology
　　g. Hysterosalpingography to assess tubular patency
　　h. Culdoscopy to assess tubular function
　　i. Laparoscopy to view pelvic organs directly
　　j. BASAL BODY TEMPERATURE monitoring
　　k. Menstrual cycle mapping to track ovulatory and anovulatory cycles for 6 months
　　l. Endometrial biopsy to assess cyclic development of endometrium
　2. Male
　　a. Urologic, medical, sexual, surgical, and occupational history
　　b. Physical examination
　　c. Review of personal habits, including medications, use of tobacco and alcohol, clothing, and bathing
　　d. Laboratory examinations: spermatozoa analysis, complete blood count, urinalysis, sedimentation rate, and hormonal testing, such as LH, FSH, and testosterone
E. Emotional reactions to infertility
　1. The couple may demonstrate behaviors associated with loss: surprise, denial, anger, bargaining, depression, and finally acceptance
　2. Infertility can lower self-esteem and elicit feelings of inadequacy, loss of control over life, and rejection by society
　3. Medical investigations into infertility lead to embarrassment, decreased privacy, and disruption of normal, spontaneous sexual relations
　4. The infertile couple who ultimately conceives may exhibit the normal ambivalence associated with pregnancy (see Chapter 4, III, A)
F. Management of infertility
　1. Surgical management: correction of anatomic defects and removal of obstructions in the reproductive tract

2. Medications used when infertility is caused by anovulation
   a. Clomiphene (Clomid) for hypothalamic suppression
   b. Bromocriptine (Parlodel) for increased prolactin levels
   c. Levothyroxine (Synthroid) for hypothyroidism
   d. Menotropins (Pergonal) for hypogonadotropic amenorrhea
3. Medications used when infertility is caused by hormonal disorders
   a. Conjugated estrogen (Premarin) and medroxyprogesterone (Provera) for hypoestrogenic states
   b. Hydroxyprogesterone (Duralutin) for luteal phase defects
4. Medications used with the male
   a. Testosterone enanthate (Delatestryl) and testosterone cypionate (Depo-Testosterone) to stimulate virilization
   b. Chorionic gonadotropin (Pregnyl) to virilize a hypogonadotropic male and to restore spermatogenesis
   c. Menotropins (Pergonal) to aid human chorionic gonadotropin in completing spermatogenesis
5. Options for the infertile couple
   a. To fulfill their desire to become parents, an infertile couple may choose from a variety of alternatives
      (1) ARTIFICIAL INSEMINATION
      (2) IN VITRO FERTILIZATION (IVF)
      (3) SURROGATE MOTHERING
      (4) GAMETE INTRAFALLOPIAN TUBE TRANSFER (GIFT)
      (5) ZYGOTE INTRAFALLOPIAN TUBE TRANSFER (ZIFT)
      (6) Adoption
   b. Many legal and ethical ramifications are associated with artificial insemination, in vitro fertilization, and surrogate mothering
   c. The advances in technology have improved success rates for IVF, GIFT, and ZIFT
   d. However, the financial costs for many of these alternatives is very high
   e. The decreased social stigma of out-of-wedlock pregnancies has drastically reduced the number of infants available for adoption

POINTS TO REMEMBER

♦ Dominant genes produce observable traits, whereas recessive genes produce unseen traits.

♦ Genetic disorders can be detected during preconception testing and during prenatal and postdelivery periods.

♦ To provide comprehensive nursing care, the nurse must understand basic genetic concepts.

♦ Individual patient response to reproductive issues may vary greatly.

♦ The nurse must examine own personal beliefs and attitudes when facing a reproductive issue.

♦ Infertility may lower self-esteem and strain the couple's relationship.

♦ The nurse must be sensitive to the invasion of privacy that accompanies reproductive issues and concerns.

♦ Infertility can occur even after a patient has given birth (secondary infertility).

STUDY QUESTIONS

To evaluate your understanding of this chapter, answer the following questions in the space provided; then compare your responses with the correct answers in Appendix B, page 176.

1. How does an autosomal-dominant inheritance disorder differ from an autosomal-recessive inheritance disorder? _____

_____

_____

2. What are the indications for prenatal testing for genetic disorders? _____

_____

_____

3. What are the common parental responses to the diagnosis of a genetic disorder?_____

_____

_____

4. What is the role of the nurse in family planning? _____

_____

_____

5. How do the following methods of contraceptives prevent pregnancy: barrier and natural methods, hormonal contraceptives, intrauterine devices, and coitus interruptus? _____

_____

_____

6. What are common emotional responses to an elective abortion? _____

_____

_____

7. What are the three types of infertility? _____

_____

_____

8. Which diagnostic test is performed to assess spermatozoa mobility and morphology? _____

_____

_____

9. When infertility is caused by anovulation, which medications might the doctor prescribe? _____

_____

_____

10. How does gamete intrafallopian tube transfer differ from in vitro fertilization? _____

_____

_____

CRITICAL THINKING AND APPLICATION EXERCISES

1. Create a chart comparing and contrasting the various types of genetic disorders.

2. Develop a patient instruction sheet using:
   – Hormonal contraceptive
   – Basal body temperature method
   – Diaphragm.

3. Care for a couple being evaluated for infertility. Evaluate their feelings, concerns, and responses. Develop a patient-specific plan of care, including any needs for support, education, and follow-up.

4. Interview the parents involved with adopting a child. Prepare a class presentation describing the couple's decision to adopt and their experiences.

Glossary

Aberration—deviation from what is typical or normal

Adnexal area—accessory parts of the uterus, ovaries, and fallopian tubes

Analgesic—pharmacologic agent that relieves pain without causing unconsciousness

Anesthesia—use of pharmacologic agents to produce partial or total loss of sensation, with or without loss of consciousness

Artificial insemination—mechanical deposition of donor's or partner's spermatozoa at the cervical os

Basal body temperature—temperature when body metabolism is at its lowest, usually below 98° F (36.7° C) before ovulation and above 98° F after ovulation

Bishop score—method of assessing cervical dilation, effacement, station, consistency, and position to determine readiness for induction of labor

Conduction—loss of body heat to a solid, cooler object through direct contact

Congenital disorder—disorder present at birth that may be caused by genetic or environmental factors

Convection—loss of body heat to cooler ambient air

Corpus luteum—yellow structure, formed from a ruptured graafian follicle, that secretes progesterone during the second half of the menstrual cycle; if pregnancy occurs, the corpus luteum continues to produce progesterone until the placenta assumes that function

Cotyledon—one of the rounded segments on the maternal side of the placenta, consisting of villi, fetal vessels, and an intervillous space

Cryptorchidism—undescended testes

Cul-de-sac—pouch formed by a fold of the peritoneum between the anterior wall of the rectum and the posterior wall of the uterus; also known as Douglas' cul-de-sac

Dilation—widening of the external cervical os

Doll's eye phenomenon—movement of a neonate's eyes in a direction opposite to which the head is turned; this reflex typically disappears after 10 days of extrauterine life

Dystocia—difficult labor

Effacement—thinning and shortening of the cervix

Embryo—conceptus from the time of implantation to 5 to 8 weeks

Endometrium—inner mucosal lining of the uterus

Epstein's pearls—small white firm epithelial cysts on the neonate's hard palate

Evaporation—loss of body heat when fluid on the body surface changes to a vapor

Fetus—conceptus from 5 to 8 weeks until term

Follicle-stimulating hormone—hormone produced by the anterior pituitary gland that stimulates the development of the graafian follicle

Gamete intrafallopian tube transfer—placement of ovum and spermatozoa into the end of the fallopian tube via laparoscope; also called in vivo fertilization

General anesthesia—use of pharmacologic agents to produce loss of consciousness, progressive central nervous system depression, and complete loss of sensation

Hematoma—collection of blood in the soft tissue

Hereditary disorder—disorder passed from one generation to another

Heterozygous—presence of two dissimilar genes at the same site on paired chromosomes

Homans' sign—calf pain on leg extension and foot dorsiflexion; an early sign of thrombophlebitis

Homozygous—presence of two similar genes at the same site on paired chromosomes

Informed consent—written consent obtained by the doctor after the patient has been fully informed of the planned treatment, potential side effects, and alternative management choices

In vitro fertilization—fertilization of an ovum outside the woman's body, followed by reimplantation of the blastocyte into the woman

Involution—reduction of uterine size after delivery; may take up to 6 weeks

Lecithin and sphingomyelin—phospholipids (surfactants) that reduce surface tension and increase pulmonary tissue elasticity

Leukorrhea—white or yellow vaginal discharge

Local anesthesia—blockage of sensory nerve pathways at the organ level, producing loss of sensation only in that organ

Lochia—discharge after delivery from sloughing of the uterine decidua

Luteinizing hormone—hormone produced by the anterior pituitary gland that stimulates ovulation and the development of the corpus luteum

Molding—shaping of the fetal head caused by shifting of sutures in response to pressure exerted by the maternal pelvis and birth canal during labor and delivery

Myometrium—middle muscular layer of the uterus made up of three layers of smooth, involuntary muscles

Neonate—an infant between birth and the 28th day

Nevus pilosus—"hairy nerve"; dermal sinus at the base of the spine, commonly associated with spina bifida

Oligohydramnios—severely reduced and highly concentrated amniotic fluid

Ovum—conceptus from time of conception until primary villi appear, approximately 4 weeks after the last menstrual period

Perimetrium—outer serosal layer of the uterus

Polyhydramnios—abnormally large amount (more than 2,000 ml) of amniotic fluid in the uterus

Puerperium—interval between delivery and 6 weeks after delivery

Radiation—loss of body heat to a solid cold object without direct contact

Regional anesthesia—blockage of large sensory nerve pathways in an organ and its surrounding tissue, producing loss of sensation in that organ and in the surrounding region

Semen—white, viscous secretion of the male reproductive organs that consists of spermatozoa and nutrient fluids ejaculated through the penile urethra

Station—relationship of the presenting part to the ischial spines

Strabismus—condition characterized by imprecise muscular control of ocular movement

Subinvolution—failure of uterus to return to normal size following delivery

Surrogate mothering—conceiving and carrying a pregnancy to term with the expectation of turning the infant over to contracting, adoptive parents

Tocolytic agent—medication that stops premature contractions

Zygote intrafallopian tube transfer—fertilization of the ovum outside the mother's body, followed by reimplantation of the zygote into the fallopian tube via laparoscope

Answers to Study Questions

CHAPTER 1

1. The family structure has changed from a nuclear one to formats composed of various participants, such as single-parent, blended, cohabitating, and extended.
2. Families may negatively influence a pregnancy if the mother is very young or if the pregnancy was unplanned. Supportive family members can positively influence the pregnancy by helping to meet the woman's physical and psychosocial needs.
3. The pregnant patient and her family can receive care in outpatient settings (such as a clinic), in an inpatient acute care hospital, or in a birthing center.
4. The nurse must explore her own beliefs and present a nonjudgmental attitude, even if she disagrees with a patient's decision (for example, on abortion).

CHAPTER 2

1. The labia minora unite to form the fourchette.
2. The uterus receives support from the broad, round, and uterosacral ligaments.
3. The female reproductive cycle consists of the menstrual, proliferative, secretory, and ischemic phases.

CHAPTER 3

1. The male gamete is produced in the seminiferous tubules of the testes; the female gamete is produced in the graafian follicle of the ovary.
2. After the morula enters the uterus, a cavity then forms within the dividing cells, thus changing the morula into a blastocyst.
3. After implantation, the endometrium is called the decidua.
4. The two fetal membranes are the chorion and amnion.
5. Placental function depends on maternal circulation.

CHAPTER 4

1. Probable signs of pregnancy include uterine enlargement, Goodell's sign, Chadwick's sign, Hegar's sign, Braxton-Hicks contractions, ballottement, and positive pregnancy test results.
2. Displacement of the diaphragm elevates the heart upward and to the left.
3. Common psychological responses to pregnancy include ambivalence, acceptance, introversion, and emotional lability.
4. The nurse should instruct the patient with breast tenderness and enlargement to wear a well-fitting support bra.

5. Common discomforts of the second and third trimesters include heartburn, hemorrhoids, constipation, backache, leg cramps, shortness of breath, and ankle edema.

6. Nägele's rule determines the estimated date of delivery by subtracting 3 months from the first day of the last menstrual period and adding 7 days.

7. A reactive NST is interpreted as two or more FHR accelerations of 15 beats/minute that occur within 20 minutes and that last at least 15 seconds.

8. The five biophysical variables are fetal breathing movements, body movements, muscle tone, amniotic fluid volume, and fetal heart rate reactivity.

CHAPTER 5

1. Factors that may place a woman at increased risk of a high-risk pregnancy include maternal age, parity, presence of chronic/acute medical conditions, and past obstetric history.

2. Three signs of PIH are edema, elevated blood pressure, and proteinuria.

3. A woman diagnosed as having an incompetent cervix will have a purse string suture, called a cerclage, placed in her cervix to help keep it closed.

CHAPTER 6

1. During the active phase of the first stage of labor, cervical dilation measures from 4 to 7 cm. Moderate to strong contractions are approximately 5 to 8 minutes apart and last 45 to 60 seconds. The mother becomes serious and concerned about the progress of labor and may ask for pain medication or use breathing techniques.

2. The primary activity during the fourth stage is to promote maternal-neonate bonding.

3. If the patient's blood pressure drops during labor or delivery, the nurse should position the patient on the left side, increase the primary I.V. flow rate, and administer oxygen via face mask at 6 to 10 liters/minute.

4. The mechanisms of labor are engagement, descent, flexion, internal rotation, extension, and external rotation.

5. Labor is influenced in part by fetal head, lie, presentation, attitude, and position.

6. During labor, the mother's oxygen consumption and respiratory rate increase.

7. External electronic fetal monitoring evaluates decreased variability of and periodic changes in fetal heart rate, grossly evaluates contractions, and provides a permanent record.

8. The three phases of a uterine contraction are the increment, acme, and decrement.

9. Variable decelerations of fetal heart rate are caused by umbilical cord compression.

10. Indications for a cesarean delivery include cephalopelvic disproportion, uterine dysfunction, fetal malposition or malpresentation, previous uterine surgery, complete or partial placenta pre-

via, preexisting medical condition, prolapsed umbilical cord, and fetal distress.

11. Readiness for induction depends on fetal maturity and position and cervical readiness.

12. Methods used to induce labor include amniotomy, oxytocin infusion, and insertion of prostaglandin gel for cervical preparation.

CHAPTER 7

1. HELLP stands for Hemolysis, Elevated Liver enzymes, Low platelets.

2. Terbutaline causes smooth muscle relaxation by stimulating beta$_2$ receptor sites in the uterus. Both magnesium sulfate and nifedipine interfere with the production of calcium, which has been associated with labor initiation. Indomethacin prevents the production of prostaglandins, which have been associated with labor initiation.

3. Management of the woman with a postpartum hemorrhage include assessment for a distended bladder, checking color, amount and consistency of lochia, massaging the uterus, and administering oxytocin.

4. The woman with premature rupture of membranes is at increased risk for chorioamnionitis, while the fetus-neonate is also at risk for infection and/or perinatal mortality.

CHAPTER 8

1. Apgar scoring is done at 1 and 5 minutes after birth.

2. The first temperature is taken rectally to check for rectal patency.

3. Cardiovascular changes occurring with extrauterine adaptation include functional closure of the foramen ovale; constriction of the ductus arteriosus; and immediate closure of the umbilical veins, arteries, and ductus venosus.

4. The anterior fontanel closes in about 18 months; the posterior fontanel closes in about 8 to 12 weeks.

5. To elicit Moro's reflex, the nurse would lift the neonate above the crib and then suddenly lower the neonate; this causes symmetrical extension, then abduction, of the arms and legs, and the fingers spread to form a "C."

6. The period of reactivity begins at birth and lasts about 30 minutes. During this time, the neonate's respiratory and heart rates increase. The neonate is awake and active and may demonstrate the sucking reflex. It is an ideal time to initiate mother-infant bonding and breast-feeding.

7. Daily nutritional requirements for an infant include 95 to 145 kcal/kg of body weight, 2.2 g of protein/kg of body weight for the first 6 months, and 130 to 200 ml of fluid/kg of body weight.

CHAPTER 9

1. Transient tachypnea of the neonate can result from aspiration of amniotic or tracheal fluid, compounded by delayed clear-

ing of the airway or excess fluid in the lungs.

2. RhoGAM is ineffective when the mother is already sensitized.

3. Clinical manifestations of hydrocephaly include head enlargement, forehead prominence, "sunset eyes," weakness, irritability, and seizures.

4. TORCH consists of *TO*xoplasmosis, *R*ubella, *C*ytomegalovirus, and *H*erpesvirus Type II.

CHAPTER 10

1. During the first 24 hours, the new mother should expect to see her urine output increase.

2. Postpartum psychological adjustment consists of the taking-in, taking-hold, and letting-go phases.

3. A distended bladder can impede the downward descent of the uterus.

4. Lochia changes within the first few weeks of delivery as follows: Lochia rubra (days 1 to 3) has a fleshy odor and is bloody with small clots. Lochia serosa (days 4 to 9) is pinkish or brown with a serosanguineous consistency and fleshy odor. Lochia alba is a yellow to white discharge that usually begins about 10 days after delivery and may last from 2 to 6 weeks after delivery.

5. Breast-feeding mothers should consume 2,600 kcal/day, a 200-kcal increase over the pregnancy requirement of 2,400 kcal/day.

6. The parents should be taught to wipe the umbilical cord with alcohol at every diaper change; to report promptly any odor, discharge, or signs of skin irritation around the cord; and to fold the diaper below the cord until it falls off, in about 7 to 10 days.

7. The nipples and areolae should be washed with plain warm water after each feeding and allowed to air dry during the first 2 to 3 weeks to prevent nipple soreness; after that, daily washing is adequate. Soaps should be avoided, and creams that do not contain alcohol may be applied to the nipple and areola.

CHAPTER 11

1. Mastitis is caused by *Staphylococcus aureus* from the newborn's throat or nose, hospital personnel, or the mother.

2. Predisposing factors of a late postpartum hemorrhage include grand multiparity, trauma during delivery, hydramnios, dystocia, and the delivery of a large infant.

3. Clinical manifestations of a vulva and vaginal hematoma include: a feeling of vaginal fullness, severe vulvar pain and unilateral purplish discoloration of the buttocks and perineum, both of which may be firm and tender to the touch.

4. During the postpartum period, standard body fluid precautions must be maintained. The woman must be advised not to breast-feed in order to prevent transmission of HIV. Special attention must be paid to the woman's psychosocial needs due to long-term implications of HIV.

CHAPTER 12

1. In autosomal-dominant disorders, the trait is heterozygous and the disorder is caused by an abnormal dominant gene on the autosome; in autosomal-recessive disorders, the trait is homozygous and, because the abnormal gene is recessive, the individual must have two abnormal genes to be affected.

2. Prenatal testing is indicated for a woman age 35 years or older, a couple that has previously produced a child with a genetic disorder, a couple that is heterozygous for a recessive disorder, a couple in which one or both partners have a genetic disorder, and a mother who is a carrier of an X-linked disorder.

3. Common parental responses include apathy, denial, anger, hostility, fear, embarrassment, grief, and lowered self-esteem.

4. The nurse acts as a teacher, counselor, advocate, and researcher in family planning.

5. Barrier methods prevent pregnancy by blocking the sperm from coming in contact with the ovum. Natural methods identify signs and symptoms that alert the woman she has ovulated and is entering her fertile period. Hormonal contraceptives prevent ovulation. Intrauterine devices alter the lining of the uterus so even if fertilized, the zygote will not implant. In coitus interruptus, the man withdraws his penis prior to ejaculating.

6. Following an elective abortion, the woman may experience relief, guilt, and remorse. She may relive the experience on the anniversary of the abortion or imagine what her lost child would look like as she sees other children.

7. The three types of infertility are primary and secondary infertility and sterility.

8. A postcoital spermatozoa analysis is used to assess spermatozoa mobility and morphology.

9. Medications for anovulation include clomiphene (Clomid), bromocriptine (Parlodel), levothyroxine (Synthroid), and menotropins (Pergonal).

10. GIFT involves the placement of spermatozoa and ovum into the end of the fallopian tube via a laparoscope (in vivo); in vitro fertilization involves the fertilization of the ovum outside the woman's body, followed by reimplantation of the blastocyst into the woman.

Laboratory Values for Pregnant and Nonpregnant Patients

	PREGNANT	NONPREGNANT
Hemoglobin	11.5 to 12.3 g/dl	12 to 16 g/dl
Hematocrit	32% to 46%	36% to 48%
White blood cells	5,000 to 18,000/µl	4,000 to 11,000/µl
Neutrophils	60% ±10	60%
Lymphocytes	34% ±10	30%
Platelets	100,000 to 300,000/µl	100,000 to 300,000/µl
Calcium	7.8 to 9.3 mg/dl	8.4 to 10.2 mg/dl
Sodium	Increased retention	136 to 146 mmol/liter
Chloride	Slight elevation	98 to 106 mmol/liter
Iron	Decreased	40 to 150 mcg/dl
Fibrinogen	450 mg/dl	200 to 400 mg/dl

Normal Neonatal Laboratory Values

Erythrocytes
- 5.0 to 7.5 million/μl at birth
- 3.0 to 4.0 million/μl by 8 to 10 weeks

Hemoglobin
- 15 to 20 g/dl at birth
- 14 g/dl at 1 to 3 months

Hematocrit
- 45% to 65% at birth
- Red blood cells
- 5 million to 7.5 million/μl

White blood cells
- 9,000 to 30,000/μl

Eosinophils
- 2% to 3% at birth
- 4.1% at 1 week
- 2.8% at 1 month

Neutrophils
- 40% to 80% at birth
- 34% at 1 week
- 15% to 35% at 1 month

Lymphocytes
- 30% at birth
- 41% at 1 week
- 31% to 71% at 1 month

Monocytes
- 6% to 10%

Platelets
- 150,000 to 400,000/μl

Reticulocytes
- 3% to 6%

Glucose
- 35 to 90 mg/dl at birth

Calcium
- 9 to 11.5 mg/dl in cord blood
- 9 to 10.6 mg/dl at 3 to 24 hours after birth
- 7 to 12.0 mg/dl at 24 to 48 hours
- 9 to 10.9 mg/dl at 4 to 7 days

Sodium
- 139 to 146 mmol/liter at birth

Chloride
- 97 to 110 mmol/liter at birth

Total protein
- 4.6 to 7.4 g/dl at birth

Potassium
- 3.5 to 7.0 mEq/liter

Magnesium
- 1.4 to 2.2 mEq/liter

Blood urea nitrogen
- 5 to 12 mg/dl

Creatinine
- 0.2 to 0.4 mg/dl

Bilirubin (total)
- mg/dl at birth
- 2 to 6 mg/dl at 24 hours after birth
- 6 to 7 mg/dl at 48 hours
- 4 to 12 mg/dl at 3 to 5 days

Nursing Diagnoses for the Maternity Patient and Neonate

Anxiety related to hospitalization and the birthing process

Anxiety related to inexperience caring for a newborn

Ineffective breast-feeding related to limited maternal experience

Ineffective breast-feeding related to maternal anxiety

Ineffective breathing pattern related to adjustment to extrauterine existence

Ineffective family coping: compromised related to neonatal health status

Altered family processes related to inclusion of a new member

Constipation related to inadequate fluid intake and perineal discomfort

Fluid volume deficit related to excessive loss of blood following delivery

Altered growth and development related to perinatal insult or injury

Hypothermia related to cold, stress, or sepsis

Risk for infection related to the mother's altered primary defenses during the postpartum period

Risk for infection related to the neonate's immature immune system

Risk for injury (maternal) related to induction or augmentation of labor

Risk for injury (neonatal) related to internal and external neonatal risk factors

Knowledge deficit related to self-care activities during pregnancy

Altered nutrition: less than body requirements related to ineffective sucking reflex

Pain related to physiologic changes of pregnancy

Pain related to physiologic responses to labor

Pain related to postpartum physiologic changes

Altered parenting related to inadequate attachment to a high-risk neonate

Impaired skin integrity related to episiotomy or abdominal incision

Ineffective thermoregulation related to immaturity

Selected References

Bobak, I., and Jensen, M. *Essentials of Maternity Nursing*, 5th ed. St. Louis: Mosby-Year Book, Inc., 1993.

Creasy, R. "Early Detection of Preterm Labor," *Contemporary OB/GYN* 39(11):64-65, 69, November 1994.

Gebauer, C., and Lowe, N. "The Biophysical Profile Antepartal Assessment of Fetal Well-Being," *JOGNN* 22(2):115-124, March/April 1993.

Iams, J. "Delaying Labor with Tocolytics," *Contemporary OB/GYN* 39(11):69-71, November 1994.

Jensen, D., et al. "LATCH: A Breast-feeding Charting System and Documentation Tool," *JOGNN* 23(1): 27-32, January 1994.

Kenner, C., and MacLaren, A. *Essentials of Maternal and Neonatal Nursing*. Springhouse, Pa.: Springhouse Corporation, 1993.

Pillitteri, A. *Maternal and Child Health Nursing*. Philadelphia: J.B. Lippincott Company, 1995.

Sandelowski, M. "On Fertility," *JOGNN* 23(9):749-752, November/December 1994.

Vintzileos, A. "Amnionitis," *Contemporary OB/GYN* 39(11):75-76, 78, November 1994.

Index

A

Abortion, 5, 52, 53, 162-163
Abruptio placentae, 45-46, 47i, 53
Accessory glands, 10, 12i, 13
Acupuncture, 85
Albumin, 17
Alimentary canal, 16
Amenorrhea, 25
Amniocentesis, 32, 160
Amnioinfusion, 79
Amniotic fluid, 48, 49, 61, 81, 92
Amniotic sac, 16
Amniotomy, 82
Ampulla, 9, 12i, 15
Analgesia, 85-86
Androgen, 10, 11
Anesthesia, 86-87
Ankle edema, 31
Anus, 8, 9i, 10i, 108
Apgar score, 102, 103t
Apnea, neonate and, 127
Artificial insemination, 165
Auditory canal, 16

B

Babinski's reflex, 108
Backache, 30
Ballottement, 25
Bartholin's glands, 8, 9i
Basal body temperature, 164
Bathing, 142
Bilirubin, 17
Birth centers, 87-88
Bishop score, 81
Blastocyst, 15
Blastomere, 15
Blood coagulation factor, 26
Blood glucose, 16, 27
Bloody show, 67
Braxton-Hicks contraction, 25, 67
Breast-feeding, 101-102, 143-144, 145i, 149
Breasts, 10, 25, 29, 33, 35, 39, 137
Bulbourethral glands, 12i, 13

C

Caesarean delivery, 80-81
Calories, pregnancy and, 39
Candida albicans, 51
Candidiasis (thrush), oral, 130
Caput succedaneum, 106
Cephalhematoma, 106
Cerebrospinal fluid (CSF), 122
Cervix, 9, 10i, 25, 27, 35-36, 54, 67-68
Chadwick's sign, 25
Chlamydia test, 37
Cholesterol, 27
Chorionic villi, 15, 32, 44
Chorion membrane, 16
Chromosomes, 15, 129, 158, 159
Circumcision, 111, 141
Cleft lip and palate, 124-125
Clitoris, 8, 9i, 10i
Coach in labor and delivery, 88
Coagulation factors, 103
Color blindness, 159
Conception, 15
Connective tissue, 16
Constipation, 26, 30
Contraception, 139
Contractions, 68, 74-75, 75i
Coombs' test, 50
Corpora cavernosa, 11, 12i
Corpus luteum, 11
Corpus spongiosum, 11, 12i
Corticotropin, 16
Cortisol, 26, 27, 61
Cotyledons, 16
Cowper's glands, 12i, 13
Creatinine, 17, 28
Cul-de-sac assessment, 36
Cystic fibrosis, 159
Cystitis, 50-51
Cytomegalovirus (CMV), 124

D

Decidua, 15, 137
Delivery. *See also* Labor.
    caesarean, 80-81
    estimated date of, 31
    pain during, 84-85

i refers to an illustration; t refers to a table

i refers to an illustration; t refers to a table

i refers to an illustration; t refers to a table

i refers to an illustration; t refers to a table

i refers to an illustration; t refers to a table

About the StudySmart Disk

StudySmart Disk lets you:

- review subject areas of your choice and learn the rationales for the correct answers
- take tests of varying lengths on subjects of your choice
- print the results of your tests to gauge your progress over time.

Recommended system requirements

486 IBM-compatible personal computer (386 minimum)
Windows 3.1 or greater (Windows 95 compatible)
High-density 3½″ floppy drive
8 MB RAM (4 MB minimum)
S-VGA monitor (VGA minimum)
2 MB of available space on hard drive

Installing and running the program

- Start Windows.
- In Program Manager, choose Run from File menu.
- Insert disk, type a:\setup.exe (where a: is the letter of your floppy drive), and click on OK.

For Windows 95 Installation

- Start Windows.
- Select Start button and then Run.
- Insert disk, type a:\setup.exe (where a: is the letter of your floppy drive), and click on OK.

For technical support, call 215-628-7744 Monday through Friday, 9 a.m. to 6 p.m. Eastern Standard Time.

The clinical information and tools in the *StudySmart Disk* are based on research and consultation with nursing, medical, and legal authorities. To the best of our knowledge, this program reflects currently accepted practice; nevertheless, it can't be considered absolute or universal. For individual application, all recommendations must be considered in light of the patient's clinical condition and, before administration of new or infrequently used drugs, in light of the latest package-insert information. The authors and publisher disclaim responsibility for any adverse effects resulting directly or indirectly from the suggested procedures, from any undetected errors, or from the reader's misunderstanding of the program.

This book cannot be returned for credit or refund if the vinyl disk holder has been opened, broken, or otherwise tampered with.